BODY MATTERS

BODY MATTERS

A Phenomenology of Sickness, Disease, and Illness

James Aho and Kevin Aho

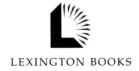

LEXINGTON BOOKS

A division of
ROWMAN & LITTLEFIELD PUBLISHERS, INC.
Lanham • Boulder • New York • Toronto • Plymouth, UK

LEXINGTON BOOKS

A division of Rowman & Littlefield Publishers, Inc.
A wholly owned subsidary of The Rowman & Littlefield Publishing Group, Inc.
4501 Forbes Boulevard, Suite 200
Lanham, MD 20706

Estover Road
Plymouth PL6 7PY
United Kingdom

British Library Cataloguing in Publication Information Available

Library of Congress Cataloging-in-Publication Data

Aho, James Alfred, 1942–
  Body matters : a phenomenology of sickness, disease, and illness / James
Aho and Kevin Aho.
     p. ; cm.
  Includes bibliographical references and index.
  1. Medicine—Philosophy. 2. Phenomenology. 3. Social medicine. 4.
Medical anthropology. I. Aho, Kevin, 1969– II. Title.
  [DNLM: 1. Existentialism. 2. Sociology, Medical. 3. Disease—psychology.
4. Philosophy. WA 31 A286b 2008]
  R723.A375 2008
  610—dc22   2008012060

  ISBN: 978-0-7391-2698-1 (cloth : alk. paper)
  ISBN: 978-0-7391-2699-8 (pbk. : alk. paper)
  ISBN: 978-0-7391-3821-2 (electronic)

Printed in the United States of America

♾TM The paper used in this publication meets the minimum requirements of
American National Standard for Information Sciences—Permanence of Paper
for Printed Library Materials, ANSI/NISO Z39.48-1992.

Table of Contents

Preface

This project grows out of conversations held over many years between its authors, father and son, occasionally beneath the night stars of Idaho's backcountry, or while free-heeling through its powder snows. What originally inspired our talk— probably underscored by the startling contrast to it of the wild Rocky Mountains—was a conviction that the instrumentalist technology of modernity harbors a profound menace. Exactly what kind of danger, we could not at first say. But its manifestations were visible everywhere, first and most obviously in the housing developments and roads creeping into the mountains with a kind of tragic inevitability, threatening the possibility of solitude and adventure. More distantly, the menace could be witnessed in weapons of mass destruction and in industrialized death camps, the global conglomerate, and the sciences of public surveillance and penology. Most perversely it was visible in what has come to be known as the "industry" of health care. It did not take us long to learn that our concern was and is shared by an immense citizen's movement that goes by many names, both in and outside of academia, one arm of which titles itself "phenomenology." To participate more intelligently in this movement and to articulate our shared problematic, Kevin became a trained phenomenologist with an interest in social theory; James, already a trained social theorist, developed an interest in phenomenology. The product of our joint pursuits is this book.

Body Matters is a truly interdisciplinary enterprise, not just an ad hoc nod to a nice idea. Both of us co-wrote and amended every chapter, ironically using (to our mutual benefit) one of the signal technologies of modernity, the Internet. Neither Kevin nor James can boast of certified expertise in the phenomenology of the body. What may at first glance be considered a disadvantage, however, may actually be an asset, given what seems to us to be the almost willful opaqueness of so much writing on this subject. In this book we have made a concerted effort to avoid the kinds of obscure neologisms that many phenomenologists succumb to. This lack of clarity often conceals and distorts the thing that is closest and most dear to us all: our very own flesh. Our hope is that this book will be accessible to any literate layperson who wishes to learn about the powerful and, we think, liberating insights of phenomenology.

Acknowledgments

Academic writing is very much a collaborative effort. Although we alone take credit for the final product, we are aware of the debts we owe to our family and colleagues. We thank Kyle and Margaret Aho for their incisive readings of early drafts of the book, their enthusiasm about it, and the recommendations they gently urged on us to make it more understandable. Ken Aho and Jessica Fultz alerted us to literature of bio-fiction that stimulated our imagination. Special thanks also go to Elena Ruiz-Aho and Charles Guignon for their unwavering support and commentary, and to Richard Hearn and Gesine Hearn, who pored over the manuscript for days and made countless suggestions to improve its accuracy and scholarship. Kevin's colleagues at Florida Gulf Coast University, especially Glenn Whitehouse, Sean Kelly, Maria Roca, Jim Wohlpart, and Donna Henry, all played vital roles in seeing this project come to fruition. Our respective universities, Idaho State University and FGCU, both helped underwrite this book; ISU, in the form of a glorious sabbatical leave awarded to James, during which this project was conceived. In addition, both universities generously allotted us dissemination grants, without which this work would never have seen print. We are especially thankful to Ariel Ruiz i Altaba for the powerful image that graces the book's cover.

For permission to reprint certain selections, the authors are grateful to the following publishers and copyright holders: Harvard University Press, for the excerpt from *The Culture of Time and Space, 1880–1918*, by Stephen Kern (Cambridge, MA: Harvard University Press, 1983); The Perseus Books Group, for the excerpts from *Existential Psychotherapy*, by Irvin Yolem (Cambridge, MA: Basic Books, 1980), and *The Illness Narratives: Suffering, Healing, and the Human Condition*, by Arthur Kleinman (Cambridge, MA: Basic Books, 1988); and Yale University Press, for the excerpt from *Introduction to Metaphysics*, by Martin Heidegger, translated by Gregory Fried and Richard Polt (New Haven, CT: Yale University Press, 2000).

1

Foundations

Preliminary Distinctions

In the first two decades of the twentieth century, a group of prominent thinkers crossed paths at the University of Freiburg in Germany, including Edmund Husserl, Edith Stein, and Martin Heidegger. They began to develop a new method of inquiry called phenomenology, out of which emerged a distinction that was to profoundly impact the social sciences and humanities: *Körper* vs. *Leib*.[1]

Körper is a reference to the corporeal body, what we are as physiological, neurological, and skeletal beings. It is what modernity's preeminent philosopher, René Descartes (1596–1650), refers to as that aspect of ourselves "extended in space," visible to the eye, and hence subject to scientific investigation. In contrast, *Leib* concerns how we experience this physical matter in our everyday lives.[2] If *Körper* is the abstract body-in-general, one object among others that is simply "there," *Leib* is *my* body in particular, my life here and now, what I am as a volitional, sensing person. It is what I see, think, and remember about my own skin and bones, and how I feel about them. To express it differently, *Leib* is the way we typically "body forth" (*leiben*) into the world, how we comport ourselves for the most part given our history and culture. Husserl and his colleagues argue that however helpful the objective metrics of *Körper* may be—that is, in assessing caloric intake, blood pressure, lipid profiles, prostate specific antigens, and the like—they are inadequate when it comes to capturing the everyday experiences of appetite, stress, chest pain, or frequent nightly urination. The scientific measurement of the body, in other words, overlooks the actual lived experience of embodiment.

The division between *Körper* and *Leib* not only affected early twentieth-century German social theory, it also had a decisive impact on French thinking, especially on the work of Maurice Merleau-Ponty, who, when he learned of it, reportedly underwent "an almost voluptuous experience" (Carman, 1999, 207).[3] Merleau-Ponty's *Phenomenology of Perception* (1962), however, represents a major shift in emphasis away from the temporal aspects of bodily experience—Husserl's and Heidegger's major concern—to its *spatial* qualities. By interpreting "my own body" (*le corps propre*) as a concrete way of living that tacitly understands the world in terms of practical movement and orientation, Merleau-Ponty recognizes that "to be a body is to be tied to a world" (1962, 148). As I negotiate a crowded sidewalk, for instance, open my office door, or get in and out of my car, my whole body is already seamlessly woven into the world. Merleau-Ponty goes on to say that this interconnectedness is so fundamental to our being that we can experience it with body parts we no longer have, as armless amputees do who "reach" for things with phantom limbs.

Iris Marion Young further elaborates on this idea in her pioneering essay, "Throwing Like A Girl" (Young, 1990; Young, 2005), where she explores differences in the way men and women spatially engage the world. An appreciation of *Leib* is also evident in the recent explosion of literary and nonfiction accounts of female embodiment, including "body dismorphia," wherein pencil-thin anorexics see obese faces staring back at them from their mirrors (Phillips, 1996), as well as the countless studies of human sexuality in all its "polymorphous perversity," beginning with Michel Foucault (1990 [1978]). The destabilization of the conceit that a single kind of sexual identity—namely, heterosexuality—is more "natural" than others (Weeks, 1991), the concepts of "emotional-labor" (Hochschild, 1983) and "gender advertisement" (Goffman, 1959), the inquiries into the "social organization" of death and dying (Sudnow, 1967), as well as disabilities studies (Wendell, 1996) and what concerns us here—the field of health and illness (Kleinman, 1988)—all have been inspired, usually indirectly and without acknowledgment, by the Freiburg phenomenologists. In fact, on close view there are few contemporary moral issues—gay marriage, women's rights, disabilities legislation, abortion, drug addiction, race relations, and the politics of aging included—that have not in some fundamental way been influenced by the simple differentiation between *Körper* and *Leib*.

A distinction derivable from, if not precisely equivalent to, that between *Körper* and *Leib* is the division between disease and illness (Cassell, 1976; Kleinman, 1988, 3–6; Toombs, 1992, 32, 35–37). While the two terms are often conflated in everyday discourse, in this book they have special technical meanings. By "disease" we mean an organic pathology as discerned from one or more recognized clinical or laboratory procedures: a measurable deviation from a standard of normal EEG brain function, for example, normal blood lipid or blood sugar level, normal body temperature, or normal blood pressure. No assumption is made here that such judgments are necessarily reliable or, for that matter, valid. "Illness," on the other hand, we take to mean a kind of nonquantifiable lived experience, not feeling well or not being considered well by those certified to issue pronouncements about the body: physicians, licensed psychologists, and so on.

It is important for the reader to bear in mind that we are not suggesting that diseases are somehow "more real" than illnesses; that diseases are rooted in biology, whereas illnesses are merely "in the mind." This is an argument made by Thomas Szasz in his controversial critique of psychiatry, *The Myth of Mental Illness* (1974). Szasz claims that apart from bizarre behaviors due to brain traumas, genetic inheritance, infections, or tumors (i.e., from bona fide diseases), what pass as mental illnesses are actually just "problems of living." We take issue with the more extreme entailments of this view.

First, while we agree with Szasz that (mental) illnesses are "socially constructed," diseases are as well. Many modern diseases can be shown to have arisen from negotiations held between doctors at annual professional conferences. Indeed, some of today's *chronic* diseases—like hemochromatosis, type-1 diabetes, high cholesterol, and sickle cell anemia—are hypothesized to have protected people in an earlier age against diseases like iron deficiency, bubonic plague, vitamin-D deficiency, and malaria. In other words, at one time they might have been considered health-promoting conditions (Moalem and Prince, 2007; Sedgwick, 1973). Secondly, what Szasz considers problems of personal living—temper tantrums, depressions, obsessions, panics, and the like—are as rooted in our biology as any other state. Each has its own unique neuro-hormonal signature. In sum, Szasz's theory betrays a commitment to the Cartesian separation of mind from body. One of the goals in this book is to move beyond Cartesian dualism.

Let us return now to the difference between disease and illness. Often, one reason why we don't feel well is precisely because we are diseased. We have a wound, an infection, or some kind of structural malformation. Yet it is also true that one can be seriously diseased—for example, with "the silent killer," high blood pressure or, say, with early stage ovarian or prostate cancer—yet feel and be considered by others, including medical authorities, perfectly well. By the same token, one may be entirely disease-free yet judged to be "sick." One of the most striking features of modern culture is the medical pathologizing of conditions that, until quite recently, were considered perfectly normal. One example is shortness, an alleged "disease" that is now said to be "treatable" by means of growth hormone injections. Another is the entire body of "ladies' conditions": premenstrual syndrome, menopause, infertility, birthing, and so on. We will have much more to say about this subject later. There are also, what are called somatoform conditions or MUDs, "medically unexplained diseases" (Hearn, 2006). These are physically debilitating conditions that are inexplicable in disease terms. In other words, they have no evident organic cause: irritable bowel syndrome (IBS), burning mouth syndrome (BMS), benign chronic intractable pain syndrome (BCIPS), and such. The last is a crippling, energy-sapping state for which, ironically, one recommended palliative is exercise, and that cannot be traced to a physical lesion (hence, the adjective "benign") (Groopman, 2000).

Related to the distinction between illness and disease is an even more important one, that between their respective complements: health, on the one hand, and normality, or between healing and curing. Again, it is imperative not to exaggerate their separation. However, it is unassailable that organic normality, the absence of any recognized biological infirmity, is immeasurably more restrictive in scope than health. "Health" suggests wholeness, completeness, and balance. It is even linguistically associated with the word "holiness."[4] Thus, while after taking vitamin B_{12} a blood test may indicate that a patient has been cured of anemia (in that their iron level now registers within one standard deviation of a medically agreed-upon statistical norm), their level of overall health may yet remain in question.

Hans-Georg Gadamer writes that health is concealed, elusive, and enigmatic (Gadamer, 1996, 112). Friedrich Nietzsche would agree. Health, he says, "depends on your goal, your horizon, your energies, your impulses, your errors, and above all on the ideas and phantasms of your soul" (Nietzsche, 1974, 176–77).[5] Among other things, this suggests that even if a disease lies beyond reach of a cure, the person afflicted with it may be in another, possibly deeper, way healthier than those who are disease free. This is one paradoxical implication of Buddhist thanatologist Stephen Levine's *Healing into Life and Death* (1989).

With his wife and fellow "death worker," Levine helps patients, but not to overcome their terminal diagnoses. Rather, his goal is to reconcile them with the inevitable. Levine teaches that true health (wholeness) of necessity entails that we embrace what completes us as living beings. And what completes us, of course, is our own biological end—our death. Ironically, several of Levine's patients, after "letting go" of their life attachments and opening up to their own deaths, claim to have been cured of their diseases. While we may be suspicious of such reports, or at least of their permanency, there is less reason to doubt assertions that they feel happier and healthier than they were prior to undergoing Levine's meditation program.

Consider another discomfiting fact: pain. Whatever it may be and whatever its causes and effects are, issues to which we return later, one thing is certain: pain reminds us of our own mortality. It is, in a sense, a prefiguration of our own death. This is what Jon Kabat-Zinn of the University of Massachusetts Medical School, a "pain worker," believes (Kabat-Zinn, 1990; Moyers, 1993, part 3).

Kabat-Zinn sees many of the worst cases, those whom his fellow physicians have given up on. Like the Levines, Kabat-Zinn's goal is not to assist sufferers in their efforts to "conquer" or "transcend" pain. This is impossible: every toxin and surgery has already been tried and failed. Instead, it is to help patients "get in close to pain" and "dance" with it. By focusing on the qualities of the pain sensation itself, again and again shelving the fearful thoughts and images conjured by it, patients become aware that much of their pain experience is a concoction of their own minds. They come to realize, in other words, that the pain sensation is not, as they once feared, "always there 24/7"; that it is not literally "killing them"; that they don't actually "have to give up everything" because of it. Fleeing in panic from pain produces greater pain, according to Kabat-Zinn. Admitting it into one's life paradoxically heals. As to critics who angrily stamp their feet and reply, "I don't want it!" Kabat-Zinn's reply is, "Well, then, good luck." To be alive, to be completely human, to be "healthy," is in part to suffer.

Why This Book

Our goal in this book is to clear a path through a clutter of stale assumptions and self-defeating ways of thinking our bodies, and to see ourselves and our afflictions in a more thoughtful way. In part what begs for this reopening is the exponentially growing expense of biomedicine relative to its proportionally smaller returns in increased life expectancy and life quality.[6] At least in advanced countries, this is forcing publics to reconsider the wisdom of continuing the present course of bigger and more. In other words, it is becoming evident that the issue facing health care in Euro-America is not just a tactical one of making the latest medical technologies and pharmaceuticals more widely and equitably distributed, as important as this is. It is a strategic question concerning the *raison d'être* of modern medicine in the first place.

One of the first books to raise this issue was Ivan Illich's *Medical Nemesis* in 1976. While it received both plaudits and scathing reviews (cf. Horrobin, n.d.), it became clear in the course of the debate that Illich's way of posing the challenges facing modern health care was much too simplistic. Specifically, he seemed to be saying that biomedicine is a zero-sum game of sorts, a matter of "biological accountants" or worse, "biofascists"—doctors, drug manufacturers, and hospital managers—inflicting their wills on masses of powerless and innocent victims: us. A similar plea can be found in the biomedical dystopias that today appear to be enjoying increasingly wide audiences.

In Margaret Atwood's *Oryx and Crake*, god-like bioengineers residing in walled compounds named for pharmaceutical companies like OrganInc Farms and HelthWyzer, and protected from the "pleeblands" by armed CorpSeCorps units, fabricate an entire zoology of new species through gene-splicing. These include a demi-human race of violence-averse, smoothed-skinned, statuesque muscle men—a legion fit for a "gay magazine centerfold"—together with multi-toned, round-breasted, unblemished female companions. To address the problems of aging and organ failure they also breed "pigoons," on which are grown replacement parts.

For Kazuo Ishiguro and his *Never Let Me Go*, it is human clones, not artificial beasts, who serve as organ donors. Conceived in test tubes, and considered as soulless "things," they are raised in isolation from the rest of society on organ-farms until the day they begin making "donations" to their "possibles" (their genetic models). Only slowly does the horror of their scientifically predetermined fates become clear.

With the flight of the gods, the disappearance of tradition, and the decline of the legitimacy of elders, Illich, Atwood, and Ishiguro suggest, medicine has become a preeminent site of menacing authority and power. What is missing from their accounts is explicit acknowledgement of our own culpability in this development; the desire pressed upon medical professionals by patients for authoritative medical pronouncements (Gadamer, 1996, 119).

As a corrective against this slant, here we follow the methodological recommendations of Michel Foucault (1990 [1978], vol. 1, 92–102). Domination, Foucault writes, is not mainly (or at least only) something that those on top have and those beneath them do not. It is neither the stuff of repression, nor is it necessarily "seized" by secret cabals from hapless others. Rather, power is ubiquitous: "It is everywhere." And it emerges from words, from *epistēmes*, as Foucault calls them, "discourses of truth." It is a product both of the forms and the contents of already meaningful social acts and practices. As such, power is not to be found "out there" in the hands of a particular class, profession, or gender. Rather, it is inscribed in ordinary conversations: in gossip, in written communications, and in nondiscursive "body-talk."

As applied to the subject of health and illness, Foucault's idea might go something like this. It is through TV hospital dramas (such as *ER* and *Grey's Anatomy*) that depict heroic struggles against debilitation, by means of staid health conference presentations, officious medical research grant proposals, and refereed articles in the *Journal of the American Medical Association* [*JAMA*], *Lancet*, and the *Journal of Medical Virology*; through their subsequent condensations as "flashes" on the latest medical discoveries on Medhunt.org, in *Prevention* magazine articles, and Sunday supplement health briefs; through "direct-to-consumer" pharmaceutical ads on the six o'clock news, and high school biology and health classes; through the "informed medical opinion" of broadcast personalities such as Drs. Sanjay Gupta, Andrew Weil, and Tim Johnson, that the following ensues: biomedicine is transformed from merely one of many ways to grasp human agony into a reality. It is reified, to use the sociological term. It becomes a taken-for-granted staple of the ordinary lifeworld. Its institutional requirements become our own personal preferences; its recommendations, our daily habits. And in this way we become its (sometimes happy) victims. The most pivotal vehicle in the reification of biomedicine is our own willful appropriation of it to empower ourselves: to enhance our individual autonomy, attractiveness, and marketability. This, by dutifully scheduling the doctor-recommended annual check-up and attending the cost-free hospital-sponsored spring health fair; by maintaining elaborate private caches of various medications, some purchased without prescription online; and, increasingly, by buying "lifestyle enhancement" surgeries.

Make no mistake, drug companies do mount aggressive campaigns to enlist new patient populations to bolster the bottom line (Moynihan et al., 2002; Shah, 2006, 36–61); and they sometimes pay physicians to serve as salespeople (Harris and Roberts, 2007). Stories about ethical outrages committed by medical researchers on impoverished minorities in America are true (Shah, 2006, 62–76, 183–84, n. 48; Elliot, 2008); and the practice continues today by contract research organizations (CROs) in India and South Africa (Shah, 2006, 10–11, 120–31, 144–63). Physician-induced injuries are in fact a major cause of death in America, and medical researchers do occasionally misreport outcomes of new drug effectiveness studies by failing to compare them against cheaper, pre-existing alternatives (DeMets and Fleming, 1996). And lastly, hospital managers, physicians-on-commission, and medical equipment manufacturers have been known to collude on projects to "upgrade" clinical facilities without evidence that these upgrades are cost-effective (Waitzkin, 1994). Such scandals provide the ammunition for Illich's exposé, to say nothing of Atwood's and Ishiguro's novels.

Foucault's rejoinder is this: To focus exclusively on such matters is to absolve ourselves of responsibility for our plight. For when it comes to biomedical hegemony, few of us are just passive victims. We are also willing co-conspirators. Every confidence game has two players: a conman *and* his or her mark. And no one can be conned unless they harbor a bit of larceny in their own hearts. In the case of health, it is a yearning for quick fixes without work.

"Discourse transmits and produces power, reinforces it," says Foucault: the multileveled colloquies in which we all participate daily. Addressing the problematic of health care, then, must involve more than simply mounting attacks against a sinister *them*. It will also require each of us to critically examine our *own* biologically overdetermined, market-driven preconceptions about the body, suffering, and death. We believe that one of the best ways to do this is through phenomenology.

Phenomenology

Although it is by no means a unified movement, since Husserl formally baptized it around 1900, phenomenology has circulated around a central motif: "to the things themselves." Let us, says Husserl, suspend the assumptions of the social world, science, and common sense, and attend first to the phenomena right before us, to what is immediately and directly given in lived experience (Husserl, 1970).

No perception, thought, or emotion—rage, jealousy, compassion, and love included—is immune from investigation by phenomenology. Here, we use it to examine health-related issues. Specifically, we are interested in how the body, its afflictions, and its well-being are typically seen, thought, remembered, felt, and responded to by three different audiences: by society in general, which understands bodily troubles as *sicknesses*; by physicians, who consider them *diseases*; and by patients who suffer them, who experience them as *illnesses*. No suggestion is made that any one of these viewpoints is necessarily "truer" than the others. Rather, each discloses certain aspects of ailing flesh, while simultaneously blinding us to others.

In its purest form, phenomenology seeks only to *describe* how things concretely manifest or reveal themselves to people. It rarely *explains* why the phenomena are as they are. Nevertheless, in order to flesh out phenomenological accounts, it often helps to speculate on the historical/cultural circumstances out of which a particular experience emerges; the milieu, so to say, that can be said to have allowed it to show up as it does, if not to have strictly caused it. While he uses the term differently than we do here, Husserl writes of this as "genetic phenomenology" (Husserl, 1977, 175f). So, for example, later when we deal with the thing known as "disease," we try to situate it in the institutional setting believed to have encouraged its coming to be.

Again, when we deal with the epidemic of "hurry sicknesses" in chapter 3, we discuss technologies such as mechanical clocks, cell phones, and schedules that appear to have been complicit in their appearance.

Concerning genetic phenomenology, Husserl asserts that "this world, with all its objects derives its whole sense and its existential status . . . from me myself, *from me as the Transcendental Ego*" (Husserl, 1977, 26, Husserl's italics). We dispute this proposition, arguing, on the contrary, that the world is a joint project. It is not generated out of what Husserl calls the "intentional features" of a self-sovereign ego, but from our shared way of being-in-the-world, from us together as conversationalists.[7] The inspiration for this idea comes from Husserl's most celebrated protégé, Martin Heidegger.

Heidegger says that all experience is "hermeneutic." What he means is that the sense we have of anything, including our own bodies, is made possible only on the basis of a pre-given world in which we are "always already" involved. It reflects our social class, our race, our gender, our nationality, our historical era, our geographical situation, and countless other factors that need not be itemized here.

From Heidegger's perspective, I am already absorbed in a world of people, a language, and a system of morality and law, as I toss fitfully in bed anticipating my lecture in the morning. As I trudge toward campus, rehearsing my lines, I try to anticipate how "they," the students, might respond: "Should I use that possibly embarrassing example to make my point?" "But what if someone were to report me to the dean?" "The department chair told me that she might be in the audience to evaluate my performance for tenure." "What will happen if I screw up?" In short, my hermeneutic situation makes it possible for me to experience myself as a responsible, if slightly self-obsessed, professor. And what this suggests is that far from being derived "from me myself" as an isolated, sovereign ego, my "I" is derived from the world.

Later that same evening, the way my upset stomach, lower back pain, and headache give themselves to me is shaped by cultural assumptions I have already absorbed as a white, middle-class, American male. Among these is the conviction that discomfort signifies that something is "wrong" with my body and that if it is severe enough then I should seek out a doctor trained to "fix" it. Had I been raised in other social-historical settings, in other hermeneutic situations, these same sensations would not appear this way. Rather (if I were a devoted Hindu from a twice-born caste), they might disclose themselves as automatic consequences of "bad karma," that is, as inevitable results of my own earlier unclean acts and attitudes. Or, if I were a Haitian peasant, I might see them as hexes laid upon me by a local witch; if I were a born-again Christian, as divine punishment for my sins; or, as a secular cynic, as dumb fate. Whatever the case, the interventions called for would differ. In the first case, it might involve more punctilious obedience to my caste obligations; in the second, sorrowful confession and penance; in the third, a ritual exorcism; and in the last, humble submission.

One of the great boons of phenomenology, apart from satisfying our curiosity about everyday phenomena and their possible origins, is that it provides an opening, a space, for things to reveal themselves differently from what we are accustomed. By allowing us to contemplate new horizons of possibility, new ways of bodying forth, it can liberate us from the narrow certitude that things must *necessarily* be as they are. This brings us to a final facet of phenomenology.

Phenomenology is both descriptive and genetic, but when it is done well it can also be "destructive" (Heidegger, 1962, 41–49), or, to use a softer term, "deconstructive." This is because it can destabilize what Husserl calls the "natural attitude" toward the world (Husserl, 1970, 145, 151–52, 329). This refers to the conviction that the qualities of things, particularly *social* things, are naturally given and hence inevitable.[8]

When phrases like "human nature" (as in "war, inequality, male dominance, heterosexuality, etc. are just 'human nature'") is invoked, phenomenological antennae are put on high alert. Phenomenologists believe that what pass as "natural laws," "natural gifts," or "human nature," are really not natural facts at all, but social "art[i]facts," products of history and culture. Phenomenologist Neil Evernden goes so far as to demonstrate that even nature itself may be considered an artificial cultural construct (Evernden, 1992).

In this book, we phenomenologically "destroy" an extremely compelling interpretation of human flesh, one that has been broadcast by and inherited by Americans from mainstream biomedicine. It is that the body is a congeries of genetically conferred anatomical structures and physiological processes that can be monitored, and that, like a car or a washing machine, is capable of being "repaired" by various pills and surgeries. We understand that continental Europeans do not, as a rule, view biomedicine in the mechanically reductive way familiar to Americans. Furthermore, we would never want to deny that, however it is seen, biomedicine is eminently suited for curing diseases. Our suggestion, rather, is that biomedicine makes it difficult, if not impossible, to grasp two very important issues. One is the paradoxical role played by sickness in maintaining the overall "health" of society. A second is the lived-suffering undergone by the ill. Among other tasks, our book seeks to address these two gaps.

In conclusion, phenomenology makes room for strikingly different ways to talk about human embodiment. Yet no claim is made by us that it confers a definitive or complete account of the subject. We intend this book to be faithful to the fundamental open-endedness of the phenomenological project. We acknowledge ahead of time that it offers only one point of access to a thing that is always engageable from multiple perspectives. Heidegger speaks for us when he says, "whether this [phenomenology] is the *only* way or even the right one at all can be decided *only after one has gone along it*" (1962, 487).

Notes

1. Heidegger arrived at Freiburg in 1911, and began teaching as a *privatdozent* in 1915. Husserl turned up at Freiburg in 1916, bringing with him his assistant, Edith Stein. Husserl and Heidegger subsequently attracted Hans-Georg Gadamer, Hannah Arendt, Herbert Marcuse, Rudolf Carnap, Alfred Schutz, and Jan Patocka, all of whom were visiting students at one time or another. For a sample of uses of this distinction by the Freiburg phenomenologists, see Husserl (1970), Stein (1964), and Heidegger (2001a).

2. Richard Zaner uses an archaic word, *Leibkörper*. This term blurs the difference we are trying to establish here. See Zaner (1981, 35, 55).

3. In addition to Merleau-Ponty, a host of recent French and French-trained commentators have addressed the issue of the lived-body, including Gabriel Marcel, Alphonse de Waehlens, Jean-Paul Sartre, Emmanuel Levinas, Jacques Derrida, Simone de Beauvoir, Julia Kristeva, and Luce Irigary.

4. This is particularly clear in German, wherein the participle "healing" (*heilen*) is almost identical to the adjective holy or godly (*heilig*).

5. The preamble to the constitution of the World Health Organization, reflecting the open-endedness of the concept of health, defines it as "a state of complete physical, mental, and social well-being."

6. In 1900 female life expectancy in the United States was forty-eight years. It was forty-six years for males. In 1990 the respective figures were seventy-nine years and seventy-two years. Most of the increase in life expectancy is attributable to dramatic declines in infant and childhood mortality. America now ranks forty-eighth out of the fifty countries worldwide with the longest-lived populations, with an average life expectancy in 2004 of about 77.5 years. (Of the major countries, Japan at 81 years ranks first, Switzerland and Sweden tie for second at 80.3, a fraction above Australia.)

Over 92 percent of the increase in American life expectancy occurred during the first half of the twentieth century; 7.7 percent occurred from 1950–1970. Since 1970 increases in average American life expectancy have been virtually negligible. From 1970 to 2000, however, per capita medical expenditures exploded, reaching $1.6 trillion by 2002. In 2001 America spent 47 percent more per person on medical care than Switzerland, the second-biggest spender per capita in the world. In 1930, 3.5 percent of the American GNP was devoted to health care; 4.5 percent in 1955; 8.5 percent in 1985; 12 percent in 1999; and 15 percent in 2000. Pessimistic forecasts are that by 2040 no less than one-third of total spending in America will be for medical care (Freund, McGuire, and Podhurst, 2003, 19, fig. 2.1).

7. For a clear presentation of Husserlian (psychological) genetic phenomenology, see Toombs (1992, 1–7).

8. Husserl's term for deconstruction is "phenomenological *epochē*." This is a Greek word standing for the cessation or suspension of belief in the natural givenness of the world (Husserl 1977, 92–97; Husserl 1970, 256–57).

2

The Lived-Body

How is the Lived-Body?

During the Golden Age of Greek philosophy (ca. 300 BCE), the human body with its emotions and cravings came to be regarded as an unreliable source of knowledge. It was considered a realm of untruth determined by the unceasing flux of sensory appearances called *phainomena*. The soul or mind came to be seen as a substance that could overcome these bodily distortions. It alone held the promise of giving human beings access to unchanging forms (Gr. *Eidos*). As Plato said, "if we are ever to have pure knowledge of anything, we [must] get rid of the body and contemplate things by themselves with the soul itself" (Phaedo, sec., 666-e).

This disembodied theory of knowledge lingered through the Middle Ages (from ca. 400 CE to 1500), and eventually assumed definitive expression in the philosophy of René Descartes (1596–1650). Descartes is important for our purposes, not just because he represents the culmination of a centuries-old tradition; he can also be considered the philosophical father of modern medical science (Carter, 1983, 20). It was Descartes who first extolled the possibility of biopsychology, and who provided a theoretical foundation for the then newly emerging disciplines of cardiology, endocrinology, and neurology.[1]

Prior to Descartes organ functioning was routinely attributed to a variety of ethereal spirits. After Descartes, it came to be understood solely in observable, materialistic terms. Instead of being identified as a sacred site, the body was reformulated as a disenchanted, inanimate mechanism suitable for scientific investigation. Two centuries after Descartes, his convictions were vindicated by the research of physiologist Claude Bernard (1813–1878), in a series of groundbreaking experiments on the pancreas, liver, and blood vessels. Bernard showed how, like a finely tooled clock, the body's *milieu intérieur* maintains itself in a state of dynamic equilibrium, the output of each organ being counterbalanced by that of others: increased body heat by sweating, for example; fatigue, by increased respiration; and so on. Life, Bernard concluded, is not some mysterious vital force, but precisely these ongoing restabilizing processes. And death occurs when they cease.

Descartes argued that ultimately there are but two kinds of substances: immaterial minds (*res cogitans*) and physical bodies (*res extensa*), material things that occupy space. He held that because cogitation and its products do not have spatial extension, they are immeasurable. At the same time, however, being free of the sensual ambiguities and distortions that plague bodily experience, they provide the thinker with genuine access to reality. The movements of material bodies, in contrast, Descartes attributed to mechanical principles like those just then being formulated by astronomer Galilei Galileo (1564–1642), or, in regard to fleshly things, notions like those devised by William Harvey (1578–1657). After dissecting the cadavers of his own father and sister, Harvey surmised that the heart is merely a machine, a pump, not a residence for the soul, and its actions are governed entirely by mechanistic laws.[2] Descartes agreed with this; he then went on to conclude that this is true for all organs: "The body cannot determine the mind to thought, neither can the mind determine the body to motion, nor [to] rest, nor to anything else" (Jonas, 1966, 61, n. 4; Carter, 1983, 97). Rather, the spleen, liver, and stomach are but composites of (what today would be called molecular) particles. Each exudes its own characteristic particles of various sizes and shapes, which move with various velocities and vibrations, becoming manifest as gases, liquids, and solids. The perturbations of these second-level particles impinge on still other organs—for instance, the brain's pineal gland. This activates still other particles, the motions of which are conventionally known as moods, desires, and passions. Descartes believed that sight, smell, touch, sound, and taste all are products of minute motile objects hitting against what, today, we call nerve receptors.

Empiricists such as John Locke (1632–1704) and David Hume (1711–1776) disputed Descartes' belief that the cogito or thinker is the first ground for true knowledge. They insisted, on the contrary, that elemental sensory impressions must come prior to thinking. In their view, the mind is a blank slate (*tabula rasa*), passively awaiting sensations issuing from the body to be activated. Nevertheless, Locke and Hume fully endorsed Descartes' other essential point—namely, that the body is a physical substance whose functions and structures are causally determined by the influences of other material things on it, not by spirits or soul-stuff. In other words, in the hands of empiricists the term "body" came to stand for what it does today in biomedicine, a corporeal thing, or, to use the German expression, *Körper*.

It is the widely accepted conflation of bodily-ness with *Körper* that this book seeks to disturb. We do this by paying attention to the very phenomena ignored and subsequently forgotten by the Western philosophical tradition: everyday experience itself. Instead of dismissing these experiences as illusory "shadows on the cave wall," and seeking wisdom in eternal forms, essential truths, or scientific laws, we follow Husserl's admonition to attend to what is closest to us, "to things themselves": "Not explaining [them] or analyzing [them] in terms of causal principles, or even common sense, but *describing* [them]" in the richest, most faithful way possible (Merleau-Ponty, 1962, viii).

The first fact, so to speak, disclosed to me upon assuming a Husserlian attitude toward my own body is that it does not show up as some sort of biophysical object or complex mechanism. Indeed, I do not experience it as a physical substance at all. Rather, it presents itself to me as a way of being-in-the-world.

The term that Husserl and his colleagues use to designate this way is *Leib*, the lived-body, a word closely related to *Leben*, life. Prior to seeing ourselves from the abstract theoretical standpoint of physics or biomedicine, which is to say as *Körper*, we exist; we experience ourselves as alive, as *Leib*.

The second phenomenological fact is that my body presents itself to me as already engaged with the world. I am always in the world, even during those moments when I pretend to suspend my preconceptions and theorize about, say, the essence of human nature. Far from being unsullied by my place in the world, such contemplations are invariably "hermeneutic." That is, they are colored by my gender, my age, my race, nationality, class, historical era, and so on. From our first breath to the moment of our death, each of us is inextricably woven into a larger "text" of socio-cultural-historical relations. This is so true that phenomenologist Richard Zaner feels compelled to describe human embodiment as a "complex contexture" (Zaner, 1981, 98). How I see and feel about my body in the immediacy of this moment here and now; how I recall those variously humiliating or wondrous body-events in the past—my first kiss or the time I broke my arm—and how I anxiously or hopefully anticipate my body's fate in the future: all of these and more mirror this all-encompassing text.

But even this way of expressing affairs is not quite precise enough, for a third phenomenological fact is this: my body is *mine*. Not mine like my house, my car, or my dog, for, with few notable exceptions to be enumerated later, I do not typically experience myself as "having" or as possessing a body at all. Instead, it is more faithful to my experience to say that I *am* my body. That is to say, I am not usually conscious of my body being separate from me (Toombs, 1992, 51–62). This being the case, my body is not something I can be "in relationship with," not a thing I can really "own." And yet as soon as I say "I am my body, I realize I am . . . *not* my body" (Zaner, 1981, 50). For my body has its own limits with which *I* must reckon, its own pacing to which *I* must adapt. It has its own functions that go on without *my* awareness (respiration, digestion, and circulation), its own level of fatigue, its ineluctable trajectory into decrepitude and death. In other words, my body has a "life of its own," so to say, a "heft" and a "heaviness" independent of my will, and against which *I* must sometimes exert myself (for example, to sit erect or to remain still). Vice versa, I can use my body as I would an instrument or tool to realize my goals. I can cut it, cover it, and color it to foster favorable impressions of me; and I can feel a steward's sense of responsibility for its well-being. In short, then, my body is "'mine' most of all, yet [it is also] 'other' most of all" (54). It is an uncanny, paradoxical combination of opposites, at once alien and intimate. Indeed the very times when it is most other than me are precisely the moments when I experience it as most truly my own. This aching knee, for example, the knee of which I was earlier entirely oblivious, is *my* aching knee; this back pain, *my own*; this headache *mine* (55–56).

Let us return briefly to the so-called text into which we are threaded. It is first of all comprised of cultural creations, human inventions like customary ways of arranging space and regulating movement. Take, for example, the American architectural practice of positioning toilets and baths in the same room, or of transporting people by private automobiles instead of by horse-drawn carriage or foot. Or consider the way our workaday schedules are regimented by clocks. (We will have a lot to say about this in the next chapter.) The phrase "cultural creations" also refers to hand-tools, toys, cell phones, and to both licit and illegal intoxicants like Prozac and marijuana.

In addition to culture, the text is also comprised of social relations. These include personal greetings, gift exchanges, and face-saving gestures, as well as impersonal institutional arrangements like schools, businesses, religions, and clinics. It is not important for our purposes to delineate the differences between cultural artifacts and social relations. What is crucial to appreciate at this point is that the lived-body is shaped by culture and social relations. And the reverse is also true. Culture and social relations are shaped by the lived-body.

Through our collective efforts we erect our own culture and social milieu. Then, in largely unanticipated ways, these return to haunt us, either by forming us or, occasionally, by making us sick, by *de*forming us (Berger and Luckmann, 1967).

Some bodily deformations are the result of deliberation and are done out of malign intent. Warfare constitutes the prototypical example, the express purpose of which is to kill, injure, and debase "more of them than us," as it is said. At other times bodies are willfully deformed so as to comport with religious prescriptions, standards of beauty, or medical norms. Here we have in mind tattooing, scarification, dieting, circumcision, gastric stapling, and painful exercise routines—in short, what Bryan Pronger calls "body fascism" (2002). In postwar Japan young women tried to entice American soldiers by injecting industrial-strength transformer coolant into their breasts. A generation later, exotic dancers in Las Vegas achieve comparable effects by means of surgically implanted silicone. The American Society of Plastic and Reconstructive Surgery considers this a "cure" for small breasts, "deformities" that are "really a disease" (Goodman, 1998).

As interesting as these examples are, the most telling body deformations are inadvertent. They are incidental consequences of practices and interactions undertaken for other purposes. Corporate magnates do not build coal plants for the purpose of sickening people. Rather, the attendant pollution and emphysema, asthma, and lung cancer are (to use the jargon of economists) "negative externalities." They are public costs over and above the debits that companies post to their ledger accounts. This argument can also be applied to automobiles and paved streets. Americans don't build cars and roads in order to kill forty thousand of their fellow citizens annually or to willfully maim hundreds of thousands of others. The deaths and disablements are (to use a military euphemism) "collateral damage," costs incident to promoting rapid transportation. The reader can think their own way through issues like the "manly man" American diet of marbled red meat and the production of heart disease, or high-adrenaline recreations and the predictable bone fractures and paralyses.

Culture, in this regard, can form and deform us in the transparently obvious ways just cited, or with unseen subtlety. Consider placebos and nocebos.

Placebos and Nocebos

"Placebo" comes from the Latin *placere*, which means to please. It is a medicinally inert substance, usually a pill, or a neutral activity that resembles a medical procedure, but is in fact not (Shapiro, 1960). Placebos are routinely prescribed to those who are ill, but who exhibit no discernible disease, in the sense of having no physical abnormality. They are also used to treat distress arising from conditions for which there is no present cure, like Parkinson's disease or rheumatoid arthritis. Studies show that placebos actually reduce pain in those with benign chronic intractable pain syndrome (BCIPS) (Moerman, 2002, 4, 105–6). These benefits are not attributable merely to the suggestibility of naïve patients. Researchers have determined that placebos actually stimulate the brain to produce its own soothing opiates, and that this biochemical action can be blocked by substances like naloxone. (Naloxone is an anti-opiate commonly administered to patients who take pleasure in mutilating themselves.) PET (positron emission tomography) scans show that an area of the brain known as the rostral anterior cingulate cortex plays an important role in the production of these opiates. As one enthusiastic scientist says, "our brain is on drugs. It's on our own drugs" (Guterman, 2005, A13).

In one experiment, the chests of patients with angina were cut open while they were under anesthesia. They were then sewn back up without any other services performed. Postoperative self-reports indicate that those who received this sham surgery were helped as much as those who underwent full heart bypasses. An episode from the PBS series "Healing and the Mind" concerning a lupus-stricken teenager named Marette, is also illustrative (Moyers, 1993, part 2). Because the side effects of the steroids used to treat her were considered so dangerous, her physician believed that a placebo had to be devised that would allow her to be weaned off them without their benefit being lost. The consulting psychologist came up with an unforgettably repellant concoction to be taken in conjunction with the steroids. After repeated spoonfuls, Marette's immune system learned to

associate the steroids with the placebo so that, like Pavlov's sali-
vating dog, sipping the placebo itself came to generate the same
medicinal effect as the steroids. Because the "mind is in the cell,"
the narrator rather poetically concludes, Marette's mind and
body were able "talk" to each other. Whether the same "conver-
sation" would occur were the placebo administered by someone
other than a lab-coated professional is an open question.

The placebo effect is so widely acknowledged that drug effectiveness studies conducted under auspices of the Food and
Drug Administration are now required to control for it, even
when such controls are not always feasible nor ethical (Shah,
2006, 18–35). For instance, to determine the comparative effectiveness of niacin and statin drugs in treating high cholesterol, it
is important that subjects not know which drug they are taking.
However, because niacin produces hot flashes and itching and
statin drugs do not, this is sometimes difficult to achieve. To
eliminate the placebo effect of the niacin, those prescribed with
statin drugs are given a substance that also produces hot flashes
(or aspirin is provided to those taking the niacin to counteract
hot flashes) (Kos Pharmaceuticals, 2006).[3]

The placebo effect is not limited just to pills and surgeries. It
is now evident that for Euro-Americans, the doctor's vestments
and diplomas, the antiseptic odor and spic-and-span appearance
of the office, its vials, syringes, and scalpels—the very accou-
trements of the clinic—plus the physician's brisk manner and
professional bearing can all help release our own natural body
opiates into the bloodstream (Cassell, 1991, 119–22). In other
words, just going to the doctor, or even making an appointment
to do so, can make us feel better. For people of other cultures,
however, this might not be true. Upon stepping into the same
clinic, they may be filled with dread and made worse off (Pogge,
1963). To experience comparable benefits, they would have to access a different healing enterprise, one with its own culturally
specific costumes, incantations, and paraphernalia. In short, the
placebo effect is made possible by a particular hermeneutic context, a cultural-historical background of assumptions so familiar
as to be invisible (Heidegger, 1962, 99). All of which raises the
subject of nocebos (from the Latin *nocere* = to harm).

Nocebos are body practices invested by people with negative meanings and that therefore can hurt, injure, and sometimes even kill those who undergo them: witchcraft, voodoo curses, evil eyes, and so on (Lester, 1972). Placebos appear to excite the sympathetic nervous system, upping the pulse, increasing blood pressure, and releasing glycogen stores to the muscles. While these physiological responses can have survival benefits, at least in the short run, nocebos seem to be implicated in the reverse process. This is technically known as parasympathetic rebound, during which the body calms itself, sometimes to the point of death. Physicians use this concept to explain how soldiers can die in battle without ever being wounded, or why it is that spouses sometimes succumb to heartbreak following the death of their husband or wife. In 1936, a Hindu prisoner of the British was sentenced to death. He was then given the choice of being either hanged or "ex-sanguinated," having his blood slowly, painlessly drained. Agreeing to the latter, he was blindfolded, strapped to a bed, and his arms and legs lightly scratched. Water buckets were then affixed to the bedposts, drip pans placed below them, and a sham blood draining commenced, first loudly and rapidly, then slowing. "As the dripping of water stopped, the healthy young man's heart stopped also. He was dead, having lost not a drop of blood" (Sones and Sones, 2006).

The toxic effects of nocebos are by no means restricted to esoteric events like this. In his study of death and dying in modern hospitals, David Sudnow (1967) shows how the simple issuance of the judgment, "s/he is dying," can serve as a self-confirming prophecy, precipitating the physical demise of the unfortunate patient upon whom it is bestowed. Once the pronouncement is made, Sudnow observes, "social death" ensues. Nurses no longer change the bedsheets; they fail to provide water; forget meals and drug regimens; family members stop visiting and stop insisting that the staff do its jobs; calls for help go unheeded. After all, the nurses ask, what's the use? "S/he's dying anyway." No wonder that Ivan Illich accuses modern medicine of dabbling in "black magic" (1976, 107f). For when a witch doctor casts a spell on a scapegoat, the victim is transmogrified into a carrier of the void. They become something to be *a*voided for fear of contamination. They become excommunicates, "dead to the community." Soon thereafter they are physically dead.

A New Language of Mind/Body

All living things are in dialogue with their surroundings. They are not only impacted by their local geographies, climates, plant communities, and fellow creatures; they also transform these to suit their tastes. This is also true of human beings. Yet human beings relate to their habitats in a manner qualitatively different from that of other species (Hewitt, 1991, 33–41). First of all, human beings have eminently more mastery over their environs than other animals. For good reasons more and more experts agree that we are responsible for the atmospheric warming now threatening the existence of so many non-human life forms. Second, the human response to their surroundings is typically mediated by the culturally contrived (symbolic) meanings its stimuli have for them. This has two major implications. One is that while the responses of other animals to the environment are largely direct and immediate, the human response is normally indirect and delayed, sometimes for hours, occasionally for months, if not years. Another implication is that while insects, reptiles, and simpler mammals are driven to behave in preprogrammed, "instinctual," ways when presented with certain stimuli, the human reaction is highly variable and unpredictable. This is why Heidegger says of human beings that we are in "comportment" (*Verhalten*) with our world, whereas other animals are "held captive" by theirs (Heidegger, 1995, 237). For Heidegger, *Verhalten* refers, among other things, to the practical capacity we have to pause or restrain ourselves in the presence of a stimulus, reflect on its significance relative to our concerns, and only then rouse ourselves to act toward it.

Finally, we suggest that human beings are as acutely attuned, if not more so, to their surroundings as other lifeforms. We are remarkably sensitive and "respondable," not just to our natural surroundings, but also to each other. An eyebrow lifted just so to an offhand comment—one completely unsensed by other lifeforms—can silence a speaker, perhaps permanently. A smiling nod from the same auditor can elicit glee. Slight differences in the sheerness, color tone, and positioning of a particular garment—differences that other animals blithely ignore—can become a matter of momentous debate for human beings. So can barely detectable human scents, hairstyles, slight differences in skin melanin, or the width of one's nose bridge. In Hindu orthodoxy, a major signifier of one's caste or alleged purity is nose width. In 1994 the Tutsis and Hutus of Rwanda murdered one another with impunity over this seemingly trivial marker of difference. Slight nuances in musical rhythm, harmony, chord progression, and sonic-intensity are known to elicit wide variations in mood. So can virtually imperceptible voice inflections. For your mother to say with concern, "*you're* hot," is one thing. For friends to agree, "You're *Hot*!" is quite another. An otherwise immeasurable thought bubble can keep one awake for nights on end. Then the wakefulness itself can become an object of insomniac disturbance. Indeed, human beings are so deeply responsive to their external (as well as internal) environments that there is a serious question of where exactly we begin and end. What in fact *is* my personal extension in the world? What are the limits, so to say, of my body?

The classic answer to this question was first announced by Descartes. The "I," he says, extends no further than the skin-sack that contains it. Each thinker, each *ego cogito*, is encapsulated in its own private body. Phenomenology offers a different answer. It is able to do this because it begins from an entirely different standpoint. Specifically, it suspends the Cartesian concern with *what* our presumed composite substance(s) are—that is, immaterial mind and material body. Instead, it inquires into *how* we are engaged participants in a shared world. This, phenomenology believes, is given to us directly through our own bodily experience. Martin Heidegger says it this way: "whether [human beings are] 'composed of' the physical, psychic, [or] spiritual and how these realities are to be determined is here left completely unquestioned. . . . What is to be determined is . . . [our] *way to be, . . . the how of [our] being and the character of this how*" (Heidegger, 1985, 154).

Heidegger's word for the "how of our being" is *Dasein* (from *da* = there + *Sein* = being), "being there." This is a colloquial German expression that refers to everyday human existence. Heidegger uses it to underscore the fact that to be human is to be always "there" in-a-world. He then goes on to say that the how of *Dasein* is "ecstatic" (Heidegger, 1982, 267). Ecstasy, to Heidegger, has nothing to do with momentary emotional elation. Quite the opposite; he traces the term back to the Greek expression *ek-statikon*, which means "stepping-outside-self," a term closely affiliated with "existence" (267). The suggestion here is that human beings are not like desks, cars, fruit, or clothing. Rather, we *ex-sist*. We "stand-outside" ourselves. That is to say, for the most part we live "beyond our skins" in a state of incessant openness to the world, and we are inescapably carried away by it. We are not self-encapsulated egos, fearfully looking out of eyeholes cut in our dermal wrappings, doubting whether other egos really exist. Instead, we are regions or "fields" of mutual care and concern, tightly woven together into a shared text of social practices, organizations, and material artifacts (Barrett, 1962, 217–18).

Being Beyond Our Skins

There is tantalizing, albeit suggestive, support for the proposition that the human being is characteristically ecstatic: auras, for example. These are energy fields allegedly emitted by all living things, including people, that can, with proper training, be seen, and (by means of Kirlian techniques) photographed (Liberman, 1990). In addition to this is a procedure known as therapeutic touch, wherein the healer supposedly alleviates the patient's "internal obstructions," not by massaging their muscles and joints, but by moving their hands gracefully through the patient's personal "force field" (Bruce, 2003).

Whether or not auras actually "exist" or therapeutic touch really "works" are highly controversial issues in academia (Krieg, 2000). Far less contentious is the experience of sympathy, our non-conscious capacity to immediately (that is, without thinking) respond to each other's physicality. Sympathy can either be "negative," as in compassion (= suffering with another, "feeling their pain"), or it can be positive, as when we are joyously "in tune" with another person musically or "in the flow" with them sexually or while engaged in team sports. Nineteenth-century German philosopher Arthur Schopenhauer (1965) and twentieth-century phenomenologist Max Scheler (1958) based their entire systems of ethics on the experience of sympathy. Both consider sympathy a primal, unlearned, preconscious act of recollection, in which our shared flesh, our common body, the *Wir* (= We [Scheler]) is momentarily "remembered," as opposed to being dismembered.

Still another, admittedly controversial, suggestion that we are for the most part ex-statically beyond our skins is the phenomenon of prayer healing, as reported by internist Larry Dossey (Dossey, 1993). Dossey cites laboratory experiments that appear to demonstrate the efficacy of both directed local and "telosomatic" (distant body) prayer on diseased plants and animals, and in the treatment of human skin wounds, hypertension, asthma, epilepsy, leukemia, migraine headaches, and postoperative pain. In many cases the findings are statistically significant beyond the range of one chance in ten thousand. (Serious questions exist concerning the use of proper controls in these studies.)

The most telling testimonials for the proposition of our ecstatic being concern the pivotal importance of human relations for health and longevity.[4] Social isolates are far more likely than their sociable and congenial cohorts to suffer a battery of serious physical maladies and to live for a significantly shorter time. What this means is that the claim that individual human life is inconceivable outside a more encompassing text of cultural artifacts and social ties is not just true by definition; it is empirically demonstrable. "We're wired to connect, our brains are designed to be social," according to bestselling science writer Daniel Coleman (Matousek, 2007). The evidence is so compelling that world-renowned cardiologist, Dean Ornish, has derived from it the following principle: love is essential for human survival (Ornish, 1998).

To support this contention Ornish cites countless studies, including one conducted at Harvard University during the 1950s. In it 126 randomly selected healthy male students were asked two simple questions: "How would you describe your relationship to your mother?" and "To your father?" The subjects were offered four response categories: very close, warm and friendly, tolerant, or strained and cold. Thirty-five years later the medical records of the volunteers were consulted. 91 percent of those who indicated they had tolerant or worse relationships with their mothers experienced at least one serious disease in the ensuing years, compared to only 45 percent who reported having warm and friendly or very close ties. The comparable findings for the sons' relationships with their fathers and disease were 85 percent and 50 percent respectively. As for those who reported having at best tolerant relationships with both parents, the rate of serious disease was 100 percent. The disease rate for those who had warm or better relationships with both patients was less than half this. These findings persisted even after controlling for family medical history, smoking, emotional stress, subsequent parental death or divorce, and the student's own marital history. Ornish concludes: "the perception of love itself . . . may turn out to be a core biopsychological-spiritual buffer, reducing the negative impact of stressors and pathogens and promoting immune function and healing" (Ornish, 1998, 34).

Similar findings have been discerned for cancer sufferers. David Spiegel, for example, claims that "friends may make breast cancer more survivable." He comes to this conclusion after comparing the longevity of women in support groups of fellow sufferers to women who received standard cancer medical treatment alone (Spiegel et al., 1989; Spiegel and Cordova, 2001; Moyers 1993, part 3; Elias, 2002).[5] Comparable results have since been reported for men with prostate cancer, and for those recovering from heart attacks. (It hardly bears mentioning, of course, that not all relationships are equally healthy. Researchers have also found that miserable marriages, for example, put wives at risk. Ironically, this is less true for husbands [Sheehy, 2006].)

One of most interesting bodies of data relating to social support is the evident fact that "worshippers live longer than those who skip services" (Willing, 1999). Although the research is still too preliminary to draw definitive conclusions from, the differences in longevity between churchgoers compared to non-churchgoers persists even after the effects of income differences, alcohol and tobacco use, marital status, and body mass are eliminated. Evidently, the blood levels of undesirable immune system proteins like interleukin-6 decrease after attending services. Nor can the benefits of religion be attributed solely to the content of the believer's faith (Sloan et al., 1999). In other words, it does not appear to matter what faith one confesses. Stay-at-homers who receive their sermons via satellite do not enjoy the same health benefits that their churchgoing peers do. What they apparently miss out on is direct human contact, or, more accurately, some kind of physical contact. For some, pet ownership seems to confer some of the same medical advantages as marriage, human friendship, and public worship (Nash, 2006).

A Final Word

To Descartes, the "I," the *ego cogito*, is an immaterial thing. As such, it is irrevocably sealed off both from its own material body and from the bodies of other egos. Minds and bodies are divorced from each other and any possibility of a successful remarriage becomes "an insoluble riddle" (Jonas, 1966, 11), an "impasse" (58), an "absurdity" (55), perhaps the biggest "scandal" in the history of philosophy (Heidegger, 1962, 249). Phenomenology rejects Cartesian dualism, partly because it poses insurmountable methodological challenges,[6] but more importantly, because it flies directly in the face of the irrepressible evidence of our own concrete experience as willful, desiring, sentient beings.

I'm not aware of my heart, lungs, or stomach as separate from my "self." Indeed, for the most part I am not aware of them at all as they beat away, breathe, and digest lunch. On the contrary, ordinarily my organs and I are one and the same. Furthermore, I don't normally experience myself as an isolated monad, housed in my own dermal container with no bodily connection to others. Instead, usually, we "flow" together without interruption down the same conversational stream of gestures and words. Like well-trained fencers, we respond unselfconsciously to one another's verbal thrusts and parries.

Of course, there are moments when I become cognizant of having a body part, say, an ankle, an eye, or a bladder. But this occurs when I can no longer count on them: when the ankle is sprained, the eye goes blind, or the bladder becomes incontinent. Precisely then, when their reliability is lost, they are "found," to paraphrase Heidegger (1962, 102–5). They become visible as objects separate from "me." But barring the case of chronic discomfort, these moments are rare.

Again, there are definitely times when I "precipitate" out of the prereflective movement of everyday life and become painfully aware of my difference and separation from you. Think of the lonely anticipation of the first date, the first day on the job, or that memorable office party faux pas. For the most part, however, I am "dissolved" in the water I inhabit with you. Each of us lives beyond our skins in a state of mutual permeability, framed by the families, ethnicities, and nations into which we are born, moving together in choreographed concert like dancers at an elaborate ball. Let us look at this dance more closely to see how its beat and timing bears on our bodies.

Notes

1. For a contrary view regarding Descartes' place in modern medicine, see Brown (1985).

2. As a point of historical accuracy, Harvey was not the first Western anatomist to conclude that the body is comprised only of matter. In his textbook, published in 1543, Andreas Vesalius displays a dissected arm in such a way as to say that all one finds when looking into the body is more body (Zaner, 1984, 63). For Zaner's brief history of the de-animation of human flesh, see 62–67.

3. It is not just amateur scientists who fail to properly address the issue of placebos. In the STAR*D (Sequenced Treatment Alternatives to Relieve Depression) trials, one of the most elaborate and expensive federally funded studies ever conducted on anti-depression drugs, experimenters failed to use a

placebo control group (Rush et. al., 2006, 1240). Thus there was no way to conclude whether the drugs were more effective in reducing depression than sugar pills (pretend medicine) or doing nothing at all. In fact, given the 70 percent non-remission rate for depressives who took the drugs during the first phase of the experiment, plus their proven toxicity, some psychiatrists suspect that they have no medical benefit at all (Sinaikin, 2006, 5; Medical News Today, 2006). This is significant given that all of the researchers involved in the STAR*D trials were also paid "consultants" of the pharmaceutical companies that produced the drugs being tested (Rush et al., 2006, 1241).

4. For a review of five studies that support this conjecture, see House et al. (1994, 83–92).

5. A follow-up study completed in 2001 did not confirm this. Spiegel gives as reasons better chemotherapy given to all women, regardless of whether they attend support groups, and the ad hoc use of support groups by women who were not formally enlisted in his personal study.

6. Thus far, all academically reputable attempts at overcoming Descartes' "mortal weakness" have taken a reductionist turn. That is, they attempt to replace mind-words like "will," "mood," and "feeling" with terms from molecular bio-chemistry (cf. Pert [1999]; McEwen and Lasley [2002]; and Damasio [1999]). Descartes himself anticipated this move when he inscribed the following proposition: "soul [i.e., the contents of consciousness] is nothing else than a certain disposition of the parts of [one's] body" (Jonas, 1966, 61, n. 3). For the methodological difficulties facing efforts at overcoming reductionism, see Hempel (1966, 101–10).

Chapter 3

The Accelerated Body and Its Pathologies

The lived-body is a *how*, not a *what*. It is a way or a manner by which we concretely engage a particular historical situation. One component of any situation, something usually so familiar as to be considered unworthy of comment, is time: the procession of events, one thing after another. The different ways that temporal processions can be lived, how they can be seen, thought, and suffered, are countless. The Native American world, for example, moves to the rhythms of "Indian time," without the insistence on punctuality that is so important for "Anglos." Mexican Americans also distinguish between European clock time and *hora mexicana*, a more relaxed and open-ended sequence of affairs. European travelers to the Middle East used to complain of "Turkish time" or "Arab time." The Turkish day was broken into twenty-four hours, but in Muslim law, the day was said to begin at sunset. Since sunset varies by season, this meant that European timepieces had to be frequently reset, frustrating efforts at coordinating joint activities (Lewis, 2002, 120–21). Muslims were reluctant to adopt European clocks over fears that they would undermine the authority of the five daily calls to prayer by the muezzin (118).

Ethnographers report that the Kapaukua of Papua abjure working two consecutive days; the !Kung Bushman takes pride in only working two and a half days per week; the Sandwich

Islanders work no more than four hours a day (Levine, 1997, 10; Levine, 2005, 355–70). In terms of our own European history, Thomas Anderson writes that

> in Medieval Europe, holidays, holy days, took up one-third of the year in England, almost five months of the year in Spain—even for peasants. Although work was from sunrise to sunset, it was casual, able to be interrupted for a chat with a friend, a long lunch, a visit to the pub or the fishing hole—none of which a modern factory office worker dare. [In this respect] American workers at the end of this century have fallen behind their medieval ancestors! Our incredible growth in technology has not resulted in a corresponding increase in leisure. (Anderson, 1997, 1; O'Malley 2005, 388)

In this chapter we turn our attention to the Euro-American experience of accelerated time and to the subject of how this both forms and occasionally deforms our flesh, producing what cardiac psychologists Diane Ulmer and Leonard Schwartzburd call "hurry sicknesses" (1996).

The Social Construction of Speed

Social theorists have identified a number of factors implicated in the acceleration of time. One of the most celebrated, Max Weber, for example, writes of how the quest to secure salvation in Protestant sects like Methodism—so named for the methodical lifestyle of its confessors—drove believers to work ceaselessly. This, he argues, eventually led to the emergence of modern capitalism. To support his contention, Weber quotes from the homilies of seventeenth-century Calvinist minister Richard Baxter, who insisted that time-wasting is the "the first and . . . deadliest of sins." Whether it is due to "idle talk," luxury, or inordinate sleep, time-wasting is "worthy of absolute condemnation" (Weber, 1958, 157–58).

Georg Simmel, one of Weber's contemporaries, focused attention on the pivotal role played by the emergence of the modern money economy in the acceleration of life. As a metric for assessing labor efficiency, as in the motto "time is money," it compels people to do more and more in less time (Simmel, 1997a).

Marxists have also commented on the speeding up of life. Instead of analyzing theology or money, however, they look at machines and the desire by capitalist magnates to increase output. The first such machine was the heavy loom. Pre-programmed to duplicate the simple, repetitive tasks involved in weaving, it lessened the need for large numbers of workers, lowering labor costs and increasing profit. Next came animal power to spin the thread, move the shuttle, and tamp the cloth, displacing the need for human effort, and after this, water, coal, oil, and electricity. In due course "Fordism" was introduced: the moving assembly line. This brought the work to the workers, instead of requiring them to move from place to place in the plant to locate a tool or find a piece of raw material. After this, scientific management of the factory, "Taylorism," came into being. This refers to the imposition on the plant floor of findings from "time-motion" studies of various steps in production. When the findings from the studies were implemented, workers were deterred from gesturing in nonproductive ways, in effect becoming human robots. Finally, the robot itself arrived, a speechless machine that requires neither lunch breaks nor rest. With each advance in manufacturing, the time it took to complete a job decreased. As a result time sped up.

At first "proletarianization," as Marxists call it, was limited to the manufacture of iron, automobiles, and guns. Soon enough, however, the logic of saving time began to penetrate the realm of middle management, in the form of advances in office technology. Quill was replaced by pen, pen by manual typewriter, and this by word processor. Paper files and rotary phones were superseded by e-files and cell phones. Dictaphones, faxing, and laptops appeared, each packaged with the promise of overcoming the impediments of geographic space. Comparable changes occurred in transportation. The effective size of the world "shrunk." The velocity of time increased.

These and countless other factors began to come together in the late nineteenth century, creating a radical break from the pace of rural, agrarian life. William Dean Howell, an early social critic, described the result in this depiction of life in New York City at the turn of the nineteenth century:

> People are born and married, and live and die in the midst of an uproar so frantic that you would think they would go mad of it; and I believe the physicians really attribute something of the growing prevalence of neurotic disorders to the wear and tear of the nerves from the rush of the trains passing [each moment], and the perpetual jarring of the earth and the air from their swift transit. (Kern, 1983, 126)

As early as 1881, New York physician George M. Beard was searching for a label to characterize the psychic impact of acceleration associated with new technologies of communication (the power press and telegraph), transportation (the steam-driven railroad and shipping vessel), and mechanized forms of mass production. He first proposed "neurasthenia." Later he coined what he felt was a more accurate phrase: "American nervousness" (Lutz, 1991, 4; O'Malley, 2005, 384). Writing at the same time, Philip Coombs Knapp applied the term "Americanitis" to the condition (O'Malley, 2005, 386). Whatever its proper name, Beard was convinced that it was placing inordinate strain on the "nerve force," the energy reserves, of his patients and would eventually lead to "nervous bankruptcy" (Lutz, 1991, 4; O'Malley, 2005, 384). This, he alleged, is a precursor to "dyspepsia, headaches, paralysis, insomnia, anesthesia, neuralgia, rheumatic gout, spermatorrhea [wet dreams] . . . and menstrual irregularities" (Beard, 1880, vi; Shorter, 1997, 130).

The enthusiastic reception of Beard's observations by Europeans, including Sigmund Freud, who incorporated them into his *Civilization and Its Discontents*, suggested that neurasthenia was not a uniquely American experience. On the contrary, it seemed to comport with what Simmel and other European sociologists like Ferdinand Tönnies were already saying (Tönnies, 1957). Whether it was New York, Berlin, Paris, or London, industrialized urbanization was producing a new way of being in the world, one radically different from the slow tempo of the rural community (Shorter, 1997, 130). The nineteenth century was becoming a "nervous century," an "excitable era," one that called for a new kind of physician, an "urban nerve-specialist" (113).

Among the changes that contributed to the making of a nervous century was something we have become so accustomed to that it is scarcely noticed. It was a shift in the interpretation of time itself, a shift rooted in the invention of the mechanical clock. Let us examine this more closely.

In his comparison of standard average European (SAE) time with Hopi Indian time, anthropologist Benjamin Whorf (1956) shows that far from being natural, our conception of time as a linear continuum broken into intervals of equal length is in fact culturally constituted. It isn't necessary to go into the intricacies of his argument except to say that this linear conception of time has encouraged a number of characteristic SAE enterprises. These include an insistence on punctuality (that one be "on point" on the timeline, as they have promised), synchronicity (the coordinated positioning of several people simultaneously on the timeline), historiography and paleontology (the exact locating of past events on the timeline), and, most revealingly, a plethora of behaviors like "wasting time" (as one might waste perfectly good food), "selling" and "buying" time (as one would sell or buy apples or wheat), and "saving time" (by shortening the distance traveled on the timeline to accomplish a task). All of these in turn imply a capacity to "measure" time (as one would measure any object with extension) by counting off seconds, minutes, or hours.

Long before the modern era, SAEs had attempted to measure time by Egyptian sundials, Greek dripping-water clocks, and hourglasses. During the ninth century, Roman Catholic monasteries began experimenting with heavy weight-driven oscillators to advance time pointers at controlled rates. By means of these clumsy devices the lives of monks—consisting of prayer, work, study, eating, and rest—could be regimented on an approximate three-hour basis: matins, prime, terce, sext, etc. Around 1550 the Protestant reformer and Augustinian monk, Martin Luther, issued a calamitous pronouncement. Henceforth, he decreed, all men shall live "like unto monks." Following this, the clock in the abbey tower was relocated to the center of the burg. Now the laity, like the monks before them, could begin regulating their affairs according to the chimes of the carillon bells. Soon afterwards, the Dutch Protestant scientist, Christiaan Huygens, devised the pendulum clock. "Speed," as we know it today (originally, "spede" or "spēd"), entered the common argot as a reference to velocity, the distance traveled by an object per time unit. This was in contrast to its older meaning as success or prosperity, as in the phrase "Godspeed" (Levine, 1997, 57; Gleick, 2000, 51). The end result was that in less than two centuries, time for SAEs had been transformed into a series of ever-fleeting "now-points" that were considered capable of being "managed," and a cottage industry of self-help books had arisen to aid them in this task. One of the most notable of these was Benjamin Franklin's *Advice to A Young Tradesman* (1748), with its "plan for utilizing the 24 hours of a day."

Today, books on time management go by titles like *Taking Control of Your Schedule* and *Avoiding Time Traps*. They can be purchased, paperback, at one's nearby "convenience store." This, to save more time, is situated in proximity to similar enterprises in suburban strip malls. Urgent Care, Quikee Mart, Jiffy Lube, KwikKash, Jet Stop, and Rapid Lab enable us "to get the most out of each moment" by cramming every now point with more and more things (Rosa, 2003, 7).

The malls, in turn, are connected by a labyrinth of freeways built to expedite traffic. Soup-at-hand in the driver's side cupholder, books-on-tape in the dashboard console, and cell phone at the ear, shoppers in SUVs converge en masse on expressway ramps, producing a uniquely modern form of congestion sarcastically known in local lore as the I-5 (or I-84, I-25, etc.) "parking lot." For ironically, "the more lanes you build," say engineers, "the more traffic you get" (Paumgarten, 2007, 65). Intending to save time, commuters increasingly find themselves "spending" it, and getting less and less in return. Happiness goes down; reports of "road rage" go up.

Skilled time managers boast of being "ahead" of time, of "getting more out of their day," of enjoying "forty-eight-hour days," or "sixty-five-minute hours" (Gleick, 2000, 231). As for the rest of us, we always seem to be "running out of time." We are constantly "on watch," glancing at our wristwatches to orient ourselves in a madly careening world, and discomfited when this bit of mechanical reassurance is momentarily misplaced.

With bitterness, sociologist George Ritzer (2002) writes of the "McDonaldization" of society—of massive clock-driven enterprises like the O'Hare and Kennedy airports or WalMart and Burger King that are organized to maximize the predictability of movement, the volume of output, and, above all, speed. Because "just-in-time" McDonaldized distribution systems dominate urban spaces, we become accustomed to them, adjust our own rhythms to theirs, and demand more of them in our lives. As James Gleick once said, prior to FedEx, when it could *not* "absolutely, positively be there overnight," it rarely had to be. But now that it can, it must (Gleick, 2000, 85).

Having little time to spare with our children before sleep, we read to them *One-Minute Bedtime Stories*. With no time to cultivate relationships over homecooked meals, we turn to the mechanized predictability of precooked Swanson microwave dinners. Or we farm out responsibility for cooking altogether—like we do our gardening, baby-sitting, lawn mowing, elder care, and now even child-bearing—to others willing to take low paying, benefitless "McJobs." With little patience to struggle through the paper version of *The New York Times*, we download its online facsimile, or subscribe to a "McPaper" like *USA Today*, with its titillating four-color news briefs. Or better yet, we don't read at all, but get "breaking news" fed to us orally in "real time" from "no-spin zones" or in the form of news "McNuggets." We avoid carefully crafted, time-consuming in-depth reportage in favor of "sound bytes." And when these impede our momentum, they are exchanged for inflammatory "word bytes": "defeatocrat," "Islamo-fascist," "gay agenda." Time speeds up; we dumb down.

Today, even mountaineering, once romanticized as a site for solitude and leisurely reflection, has turned into an exercise in speed. Self-proclaimed "world's fastest climber," Hans Florine, brags in his book, *Speed Climbing*, about ascending the granite wall of El Capitan in Yosemite in two hours and forty-eight minutes. His self-adulating web page describes "Hans [as] obsessed with speed. He times virtually everything. . . . [He] has produced an audio program [that one can attend to while driving] called 'Speed is Power'" (Florine, n.d.). It relates how Florine's college education in human resource management inspired him with a desire to accelerate everything from newspaper reading and loan closings to diaper changing and widget manufacture.

Most of us are unaware of the authority of clock-time. But noticed or not, chronometers, day-planners, and calendars not only shape our behaviors and determine our moods; they contort our postures, interfere with digestion, and pressure our hearts. This is why the method of phenomenology is so crucial. By offering concrete descriptions of average everyday ways of being, it positions us to recognize (to re-know in a potentially liberating way) aspects of living that are, for the most part, passed over unseen.

We can begin such a description at the very moment of rude awakening by the digital alarm located at the bedside table. After stumbling to the kitchen, I encounter three other digital clocks: one on the coffee machine, one on the microwave, and another on the stove. After showering, I dress, don a wristwatch, and place a cell phone in my pocket, a device that also has a digital clock on its face. As I drive to the office, I am reminded of the time by the digital clock in the dashboard. After I arrive, I see two others, one on the phone and another on the computer screen. These nine different clocks are, as Martin Heidegger might say, "handy." I am already unconsciously using them, with little awareness of what they are doing to me, how they are shaping my acts and engendering an attitude of perpetual alertness.

Because clock-time is ordinarily (and naively) interpreted objectively, as a thing—maybe like a plane or a train—that passes by independently from us, we are fooled into believing that it is possible to "lose" time. Caught up in busy everydayness, the clock tells us that we are always on the verge of "being late," that we are "pressed" for time, and never quite "have enough" of it. Heidegger warns that when we fall prey to this conviction, we risk "losing [our own personal] time." This is poignantly expressed in the familiar "I [simply] don't have time [for you, for us, for me]" (Heidegger, 1962, 377). We lose sight of a different, more primordial, sense of temporality, which we become cognizant of when we are pulled away from busy distractions and the routines of life on the clock.

In this deeper sense of time the present, my presence here and now, is experienced from the standpoint of my past and my future. By my *past*, we mean the shared historical background of practices and beliefs that influence how things count and matter to me now. By my *future*, we mean the social possibilities (roles, occupations, and relationships) that I can press into, that shape my self-interpretation, and that culminate in my own death. Taken this way, time is not something I can actually "lose," "manage," "save up," or "sell," for it is not something I ever really possess or have power over, like I do a car or a house. Rather, I *am* time, and—as a finite, future-anticipating, historically situated *way of being*—my time ends when I do.

Both Whorf's ethnography of the Hopi Indian and Pierre Bourdieu's classic study of the Kabyle peasantry of Algeria (1963) illustrate how time can be experienced, not as series of abstract numbers that signify units of length on a linear continuum, but as a shared historical context of lived events. For the Kabyle

> Time . . . is not . . . measured time. . . . [Instead] the parts of the day are lived as different appearances of the perceived world, nuances of which are apprehended impressionistically: "when the sky is a little light in the East," then "when the sky is a little red," "the time of the first prayer," then "when the sun touches the earth," "when the goats come out," "when the goats hide," and so on. (57)

Here time shows up as an overlapping series of public events whose meanings are inflected with fond memories or regrets and with future hopes or fears. It is these shared meanings that provide the background that helps orient the Kabyle to their world. To speak hypothetically, to the Kabyle that unforgettably horrible day in New York City would not be the word byte "9/11," an abstract date on a calendar, but "the day when the towers fell," "the day of great suffering," or "the day neighbor wept with neighbor."

The Kabyle regarded the introduction of mechanical clocks with deep suspicion, for it placed them in opposition to the organic rhythms of their world. Instead of encouraging an attitude of accommodation to and acceptance of life's unfolding, it was feared that the clock would turn time into an object to be mastered. This, they felt, would lead to greed and distrust. "The devil's mill," as they called it, threatened to pull the leisure-loving Kabyle into hurry sickness: haste, busyness, and "diabolical ambition" (Bourdieu, 1963, 59). "Here the sky is too blue, the sun too hot," they might have said. "Why hurry? Why do injury to the sweetness of living? . . . Strict exactitude . . . lacks suppleness, it lacks fantasy, it lacks cheerfulness, even dignity" (Lewis, 2002, 131–32).

Hurry Sicknesses

By the late nineteenth century, a growing number of psychiatrists and neurologists were beginning to address the evident increase in neurasthenia in America and Europe. In addition to George M. Beard, whom we mention above, were Karl Westphal, Jean-Martin Charcot, and William James. Among the cures they recommended for neurasthenia were hypnosis, hydrotherapy, opium, rest, electrotherapy, and psychoanalysis (Shorter, 1997).

Far from being allayed, this concern multiplied during the twentieth century. In 1959 two California cardiologists, Meyer Freidman and Ray Rosenman, published a pioneering article in *JAMA* titled, "Association of Specific Overt Behavior Patterns with Blood and Cardiovascular Findings" (Freidman and Rosenman, 1959). It reported the outcome of a large-scale study of pathologies seemingly related to the experience of modern time. In it the term "Type-A" was coined. It referred to a character structure identifiable by competitiveness, hostility, impatience, and a predisposition to achieve. James Gleick would later reintroduce Type-A personality in the form of a figure named "Paul."

> Paul hurries his thinking, his speech and his movements. He also strives to hurry the thinking, speech, and movements of those about him; they must communicate rapidly and rele-

vantly if they wish to avoid creating impatience in him. Planes must arrive and depart precisely on time for Paul, cars ahead of him on the highway must maintain a speed he approves of, and there must never be a queue of persons standing between him and a bank clerk, a restaurant table, or the interior of a theater. (Gleick, 2000, 16)

In response to an increasingly accelerated world, says Gleick, Paul's behavior and nervous system have themselves sped up. The result is "hurry sickness." Among its symptoms are "severe and chronic feelings of time urgency" (as indicated by self-reports of being up against "deadlines"), vigilance, a capacity to "multitask," and an eagerness to "outshine" competitors (Freidman and Rosenman, 1959, 96; Ulmer and Schwartzburd, 1996, 331; Levine, 1997, 21).

Freidman and Rosenman went on to contrast Type-A personality with Type-B. Type-Bs exhibit a calm, relaxed bearing and relatively moderate ambitions. They are averse to competition and display little sense of being "on the clock." The authors observe that despite the fact that Type-Bs embody attitudes generally contrary to conventional expectations, and could be judged less able, less successful, even lazy, they typically report high degrees of life satisfaction: "Most men of group B were obviously content with their respective lot in life and relatively uninterested in pursuing multiple goals or competitive activities. Few appeared really concerned with [professional] advancement, and most were far more involved with their families and avocational [sic] activities" (Freidman and Rosenman, 1959, 100).

The last half-century has witnessed an enormous amount of research on Type-A personality. Although the findings remain somewhat equivocal, they suggest that Type-A contributes directly to a number of serious physiological problems, including increased risk of high blood pressure (Smith and Anderson, 1986). It is also indirectly related to the consumption of fast food, a factor implicated in obesity, high cholesterol, and type-2 diabetes; as well as to smoking, alcohol abuse, and illegal drug use, all of which are associated with physical ailments like lung cancer, liver cirrhosis, and pancreatitis (Ulmer and Schwartzburd,

1996; Smith and Anderson 1986; Hancock, 1995). In addition, Type-A provides the backdrop for, if not the cause of, a growing number of psychiatric conditions. The latest version of the American Psychiatric Association's *Diagnostic and Statistical Manual for Mental Disorders* (*DSM-IV*) itemizes a host of new "syndromes" presumably traceable to overstimulated nerves and feelings of time urgency. Without being exhaustive, these include panic anxiety disorder (PAD), generalized anxiety disorder (GAD), and social anxiety disorder (SAD). There are also personality disorders like obsessive-compulsiveness (OCD), as well as impulse disorders (e.g., pathological gambling and shopping, kleptomania, and intermittent explosive disorder [IED]).

These and related syndromes have, over the last twenty years, been a boon for the pharmaceutical industry. Anti-depressant use has nearly doubled since 1998, with more than $13 billion in sales in 2003 alone (Sander and Colliver, 2004). By 1994, the SSRI (selective serotonin reuptake inhibitor) Prozac had become the number two bestselling drug in the world (ironically following an ulcer drug called Zantac), and it has been reportedly prescribed to more than thirty-five million people since its introduction in the United States in 1988 (Shorter, 1997). (Low levels of the neurotransmitter, serotonin, produced by pleasurable stimuli, are associated with depression. One theory is that SSRIs maintain high levels of serotonin, thus "stabilizing" the patient's moods. Another theory is that SSRIs actually generate new neuroprocessors. Assessing the accuracy of these two accounts is beyond the scope of our concern here.)[1]

The explosion in SSRI use has prompted psychiatrist Peter Kramer, author of the bestselling book *Listening to Prozac: Remaking the Self in the Age of Anti-Depressants*, to coin a new phrase, "cosmetic pharmacology," a sub-discipline in cosmetic medicine (a subject we deal with in chapter 7). It refers to medicine prescribed not to repair physiological damage, but to provide patients with what are considered desirable personality traits (Kramer, 2006, 4). In his practice, Kramer noticed that some of his patients, no longer depressed, still insisted on taking anti-depressants. This is because the drugs made them feel "better than well." They were, at least in their own judgment, able to "achieve more," be "more competitive," assertive, and alert. To say it another way, they wanted to enjoy the alleged benefits of being Type-A without suffering its psychic costs. Kramer cites a UCLA study in which employees who had no history of depression were given Paxil (another popular SSRI). They were then observed to determine how they interacted with their colleagues. None reported experiencing "severe untoward [side]-effects," yet all "tended to have more leadership qualities, be more conciliatory and be leaders in solving problems" (2).

Kramer's concern is that SSRIs are being used, inappropriately in certain instances, as a "workplace steroid." (Steroids are still another family of toxins that promise to enhance performance in hyper-competitive, achievement-oriented settings, most notably athletics.) A second occasion for concern is the dramatic rise in prescriptions for the amphetamine (methylphenidate hydrochloride) commonly known as Ritalin (Adderall or Concerta). Recommended for the treatment of attention deficit hyperactivity disorder (ADHD), Ritalin use increased 400 percent in just five years between 1989 and 1994. The growth was so massive that the U.S. Drug Enforcement Administration asked the United Nations International Narcotic Control Board to investigate. What it discovered is that 10 percent to 20 percent of all male school children in America were currently on the drug. American boys today consume more than 90 percent of the 8.5 tons of Ritalin produced annually worldwide (Livingston, 1997, 3).

A typical clinical test for ADHD is to ask a child to read as quickly as possible five rows of the letters A, B, C, D, and E, variously juxtaposed. The baseline for normal task completion is twenty-five seconds. The child suspected of ADHD takes thirty-five seconds, and then reports being exhausted at the effort. The tentative conclusion is that they lack an ability to stop their own pre-programmed actions. But "impulse control" is precisely the aptitude essential for functioning well in a world that calls for immediate responses to rapidly changing, often contradictory, stimuli. Evidently, the child falters because too much is happening. Thus, while anecdotal information claims that they enjoy video games, in fact they usually fail when playing them. It is speculated that Ritalin, like SSRIs, works by inhibiting the "re-uptake" of dopamine by the brain's receptors, making it available for cognition.

The first edition of the *Diagnostic and Statistical Manual* (*DSM-I*), published in 1952, made no mention of any disorder resembling ADHD. Its near cousin, attention deficit disorder (ADD), would not appear until 1980 in the *DSM-III* (Livingston, 1997, 7). That there was no diagnostic category for ADHD even as recently as 1960 raises several intriguing questions. Were boys growing up in the late 1950s simply more focused and better behaved than those of today? Have advances in brain science enabled us to diagnose what has always existed in children? Or, more pointedly, has the velocity of American life increased to such a degree that youngsters, say like the truant and "oppositional" Huckleberry Finn or the irrepressible Jo March of Louisa May Alcott's *Little Women*, who in more bucolic times might be perfectly well-adjusted, are now disclosed as "problems" (Gladwell, 1999, 84)?

Although there may be truth in all three of these answers and in others as well, here we consider only the last. Our argument is that ADHD (which is now showing up in adults), with its characteristic impulsiveness, forgetfulness, and jumpiness may be an unintended by-product of our own technological culture. Ritalin and SSRIs may therefore be seen as crutches that help those who in other circumstances would have no need for them, adjust to an increasingly turbocharged way of life.

Kramer does not address the subject directly, but pharmaceutical companies now boast of having breached the "last frontier" in the "war" against "lost time," a "disorder" otherwise known as sleep. Nodding off while on the job, often confused with narcolepsy, is now said to be "treatable" by means of orexin reuptake inhibitors (ORIs). These presumably interfere with the reuptake of still another neurotransmitter, orexin, making it possible to remain perpetually awake. The ORI, Provigil, has become one of the latest tools in the kit bag of cosmetic pharmacology (Groopman, 2001). With it, military pilots are guaranteed to stay alert while flying long stealth missions (e.g., from Omaha to the Middle East). Unlike the amphetamine, Dexidrine, that indiscriminately stimulates the entire nervous system resulting in jitteriness, hypertension, and an irregular heartbeat, ORIs are designed to target specific neurons so as to produce a calm wakefulness, allegedly with no undue side effects. Like consumers of SSRIs, users of ORIs report feeling like "masters of the universe!" in the words of the protagonist in Tom Wolfe's novel *The Bonfire of the Vanities*. The Department of Defense predicts that with ORIs, "operational tempo" during "rapid deployment" will no longer be disrupted by troops falling prey to sleep. This will be "no less than a twenty-first-century revolution in military affairs," enthuses one general. "[It] eliminat[es] the need for sleep while maintaining . . . high level[s] of . . . performance . . . creat[ing] a fundamental change in war fighting" (Groopman, 2001, 55). It is reported that assistant professors at leading universities in England and the United States, under pressure to publish or perish, are now consuming Provigil in order "to get that golden nugget of tenure" (Monastersky, 2007).

The possibility of a medical remedy for fatigue leads to the subject of nonprescription "uppers": energy drinks, of which there exists a virtually endless list—Red Bull, Jolt Cola, Surge, Adrenaline, Full Throttle, and Ampd—the trade names of which betray their effects. While a "venti"—a twenty-ounce hit—of coffee is the beverage of choice for American elders, their children incline toward the sweeter alternatives. In either case, given that caffeine is now being placed in everything from chocolate bars, beer, lip balm, doughnuts, sunflower seeds, soap, and bagels, it is hardly surprising that there has been a dramatic increase in still another hurry sickness: insomnia. From 2000 to 2004 prescriptions for allegedly "non-addictive" sleep aids doubled in America. It is reasonable to suppose that during that same period, usage of over-the-counter soporifics like Tylenol PM grew to the same degree. In 2006 forty-two million prescriptions were written for Ambien, Sonata, or Lunesta to help Americans "come down" from their overly stimulated, amphetamine-laced work or school days. In fact, the largest increase in sleeping medicine usage is among children and young adults (Harder, 2006, 1).

In our view, then, the predilection for speed has helped constitute a peculiar kind of Euro-American body. It is also implicated in shaping how these bodies are cared for. This occurs by privileging therapies that themselves promise speedy outcomes. Let us examine this more closely.

The major vehicle for underwriting health care in America is the managed care organization (MCO). An MCO is a private corporation that pays "preferred providers" (PPs) for services rendered. These are doctors with reputations for delivering rapid-paced, cost-effective medicine. There are different kinds of MCOs with different reimbursement policies, but one type—the type that concerns us here—favors treatment plans entailing simple diagnoses that can be entered into actuarial formulas (Cushman and Gilford, 2000, 986; Cushman, 2003). These kinds of MCOs discourage therapies like psychoanalysis, which are considered diagnostically "overcomplex," and whose outcomes are often too "vague" to measure. (For instance, a 1949 study by psychologist Philip Ash showed that three psychoanalysts faced with the same patients and given identical information on each at the same time were able to reach diagnostic consensus only 20 percent of the time [Ash, 1949; Spiegel, 2005].)

In 1980 the *Diagnostic and Statistical Manual* (*DSM-III*) operationalized the preference for simplicity and speed by introducing a distinction between axis I and axis II psychological conditions. "True" neuroses are positioned along axis I. These are restricted to conditions whose treatments hold promise of quickly reintegrating patients back into the everyday world. PPs in this case are those who can demonstrate the ability to meet the MCO target rate of 80 percent of outpatient work completed within eight to ten sessions (Woods and Cagney, 1993, 38–39). Disorders that entail longer, more convoluted treatment trajectories are dubbed "personality disorders" (PDs). These are positioned along axis II. Because PDs fail to map onto the accelerated, results-oriented MCO model, they are rarely, if ever, insured. Instead, they are characterized (and dismissed) as "problems in living." That is, while acknowledged as important in other ways, they are not considered medically treatable. Psychologists Phil Cushman and Peter Gilford may be exaggerating the consequences of this development, but their conclusion is that with the rise of this kind of reimbursement policy, the notion of personality "as an ongoing character pattern . . . simply disappears or is limited to those who can afford to have one" (Cushman and Gilford, 2000, 989; Cushman, 2003, 109). Granted this may be overstated, but it nonetheless remains true that far from promising respite from a zeitgeist of speed, some MCOs play right into it.

Speed and Depression

Let us assume that one's "up and down mood swings," their episodes of giddy elation coupled with overwhelming fatigue and melancholy, are interfering with their desire "to move forward on the road ahead." If so, advertisers urge them to "ask your health care professional if a once-a-day" mood stabilizer like Abilify might be "right for them." Naturally, they are warned that "individual results may vary." The small print also cautions that the drug may cause neuroleptic malignant syndrome, tardive dyskinesia, or orthostatic hypotension.[2] In any case, instead of being encouraged to slow down, collect themselves, and perhaps seek a deeper, health-conferring understanding of their plight, consumers are urged to purchase a pharmaceutical quick fix, an effortless way to get back on the "fast track" (Cushman and Gilford, 2000, 988).

Depression is a relatively new phenomenon. Unmentioned in the *DSM-1* (1952), it was not formally recognized as a separate medical condition until 1980 in the *DSM-III* (Hirshbein, 2006). Prior to this, of course, there were comparable conditions: melancholy, apathy, boredom, *ennui* (Fr.) *Langeweile* (Ger.), and so on.[3] The ancient Greek equivalent to depression is *akedia* (non-caring), from which Christian moral theology gets the deadly sin of sloth. This, the "noonday demon," was a familiar visitor to the cell of the medieval monk. Carrying with him a baggage of blues—weariness, stupor, and sadness—he was known to knock on the monk's door at the "Hour of Lead," during the "slanting vespertine light of late afternoon" (Smith, 1999, 62, 72; Kuhn, 1976, 43).

Influenced by the observations of George M. Beard, Simmel interpreted depression (blaséness) as the auto-anesthetizing response of an overstimulated body to sensory overload, the "shocks and inner upheavals" of accelerated urbanity that "tear . . . the nerves so brutally hither and thither that their last reserves of strength are spent" (Simmel, 1997b, 176). The *DSM-IV*, in contrast, diagnoses depression as a "syndrome," and usually attributes it to chemical imbalances, recommending anti-depressants like Prozac or Zoloft as palliatives (to lift the spirits) or the pacifying effects of Paxil. For those who remain "treatment resistant," more radical interventions are prescribed. One of these is electroconvulsive therapy (ECT); another is repetitive transcranial magnetic stimulation (rTMS); and still a third is vagal nerve stimulation (VNS). This involves surgical implantation of a timed stimulator under the skin of the chest wall to send small electrical signals to the flagging brain (Sinaikin, 2006, 4).

Phenomenology approaches depression from a different standpoint. To begin with, it does not see depression as a subjective state "inside" a person at all (Merleau-Ponty, 1962, 82); that is, a condition caused by some sort of neurotransmitter deficit. Rather, like dread, anxiety, hostility, and other moods, depression is considered to be already "out there" as part of the public "atmosphere" that I am currently involved in. To say it more directly, because human existence is always a shared, public way of being, phenomenology understands moods like depression to be disclosive of a particular socio-historical situation (Heidegger, 1995, 67).

Our feelings of emptiness at work or at home, for example, disclose the ways our jobs and marriages matter to us. They invite us to face the social choices and commitments we have made. As I cheerlessly career, clock-driven, through exhaust fumes, to "you've got mail" promptings, and "the thin metallic ping of the microwave" (to paraphrase Jeffery Smith), I am summoned to ask, "Is this what I really want to do with my life? What is my true vocation anyway?" As I approach the house after work, I am flooded with a dull dispiriting anxiety. Instead of recommending a tablet to "up" my spirits, phenomenology asks me to examine how I live my life. By keeping painful moods at bay through drugs, we may be prematurely closing off opportunities to come to grips with the existential examination of *who we are* in the twenty-first century.

Again, we are not saying that depression is unique to our era. Nonetheless many observers claim that ours is "an age of depression." Still others speak of depression as the "common cold" of contemporary mental illness (Hirshbein, 2006, 215). Today, 40 percent of American women and over 10 percent of men are said to suffer from depression. These are rates ten times greater than those just a generation ago. Furthermore, the average age of onset of depression has plummeted in the last few decades from thirty years old to fifteen years; and eight of the ten most frequently prescribed medications in the United States are intended to treat either it or other stress-related conditions (O'Connor, 2005, 12–28).

There are, of course, many reasons for these facts, not the least of which are the diagnostic criteria contained in the *DSM-IV* itself. These enable therapists to isolate more precisely psychological conditions that have probably always plagued human beings. However, it may also be true that contemporary increases in depression can be attributed to dramatic technological changes that societies have undergone in the last century. One hypothesis is that these changes have begun to exceed the capacity of human nervous systems to adapt, resulting in skyrocketing rates of nonspecific anxieties, panic attacks, and feelings of emptiness. Particularly disturbing are reports of increased rates of depression among children.

A multimillion-dollar study recently conducted by the UCLA Center on Everyday Lives of Families finds that affluent suburban kids, incessantly shuttled by doting parents from tennis lessons to fencing, and from soccer practice to tutoring, energy drinks in hand and homework on their laptops, exhibit lower levels of life satisfaction than their impoverished inner-city peers. They also report having higher rates of anxiety disorders and substance abuse issues (Verrengia, 2005). The latest findings are that diagnoses of pediatric bipolar disease (manic-depression) rose 4000 percent from 1994 to 2003. Today, they number more than the total of ADHD and autism cases together (Associated Press, 2007). Again, while we do not want to overlook the role that the *DSM-IV* has played in this surge, it is worth wondering whether the ubiquity of depressive disorders is somehow implicated in the fact that over 60 percent of American adolescents claim to know someone who has attempted to take their own life (O'Connor, 2005, 36). (Readers should bear in mind that suicide attempts are far different from actual suicides.)[4]

Social critics Ben Agger (2004) and Beth Anne Shelton (Agger and Shelton, 2007) write ominously of today's "fast families," kinship groups moving with such velocity that the experience of childhood has become an empty "simulacrum" of the hassle-free, exuberant, self-paced, and playful years of their own youth. (For Ben, it was the 1950s of pre-metropolitan Eugene, Oregon.) Agger recalls that the most up-to-date technology of his younger days was a tiny black-and-white TV equipped with adjustable rabbit ears that received three fuzzy local channels. In contrast, his own preteen children are under twenty-four-hour siege by the Internet, electronic day planners, and cell phones. As a result, instantaneity has "leaked" into their lives; the one-time honored Victorian division between work and home has "imploded." For kids of today, childhood—at least as experienced by Agger—has become essentially obsolete: "Fast families breed virtual children, kids who nearly miss childhood altogether" (Agger and Shelton, 2007, 73). Burdened with mountains of class assignments, music lessons, supervised sports, community service and church projects, like harried adults, kids labor to build resumés in hopes of accessing elite colleges, where their lives will become even more accelerated.

Heidegger would say that moods like depression tell us something profoundly important about the modern world—namely, the leveling down of all things to the status of objects to be cost-effectively managed according to predetermined schedules. Just as forests have become board feet of lumber and mountain lakes, water reserves stored up for later use, human beings are now increasingly being enframed as objects for manipulation by health and human resource management technicians.

Heidegger traces the modern experience of depression back to the Greek *Lethe*, the mythological river of forgetfulness. He claims that in our preoccupation with administering and controlling a world of beings, including *human* beings, we have forgotten about Being. We have lost sight of the mysterious historical "event" (*Ereignis*) that "gives" (*gibt*) meaning to beings in the first place. As a result, life has lost its poignancy and enchantment. It has turned into a frantic, unrelenting effort to fill an underlying emptiness.

For Heidegger the very breathlessness of our fragmented and overscheduled days blinds us to our own lethargy. In this way, it remains unthought, unseen, "silent and inconspicuous" (Heidegger, 1995, 134). In a sense, we have become so preoccupied with time-saving gadgets, so distracted by a barrage of titillations that we are unable to recognize our own depression. This, he says, is the most "shocking distress" of all (Heidegger, 1999, 79).

Notes

1. The first known SSRI, Malisid (Impramine, Iproniazid), was originally a World War II German V-2 rocket propellant. Experimenters working with it reported having euphoric feelings. Tuberculosis patients, later given the substance to fight infection, were said to have had comparable experiences. Researchers subsequently found that Malisid kept the brain from manufacturing an enzyme that broke down a then newly discovered neurotransmitter, serotonin. The inference was drawn from this that Malisid could be used to fight depression (Greenberg, 2007).

2. These refer respectively to muscle rigidity, spasmodic movement, and low blood pressure.

3. It is interesting to note that the English word "boredom" was not coined until 1768 by the Earl of Carlisle in a letter pitying his "Newmarket friends, who are to be bored by these Frenchmen" (Spacks, 1995, 13).

4. After increasing three times from 1965 to 1990, teenage suicide rates in America declined steadily from 1990 to 2003. From 2003 to 2004, however, they spiked, especially among girls aged ten to fourteen (+76 percent) and fifteen to nineteen (+32 percent). The suicide rate for teenage boys during this same period rose 9 percent (Grohol, n.d.). One speculation is that Food and Drug Administration warnings about youth anti-depressant use issued in 2002 resulted in a drop in prescriptions, leading to more suicides. For longer-range trends in suicide among all age groups in America from 1970 to 2002, see McKeown et al. (2006).

4

The Sicknesses of Society

Normality and Abnormality

From the viewpoint of society, bodily infirmities show up as sicknesses, that is, as deviations from standards that define normality and health. Beyond breaking rules that characterize normal physical and psychological functioning, sickness also disrupts routines, shatters expectations, and foments disorder. In the age of acceleration, I am already stretched to the limit because I've taken on an extra committee assignment, a teaching overload, or a promised favor to a friend. Then, uncannily, the "call" comes, usually at an ungodly, pre-dawn hour: my parent or my child has fallen sick. Suddenly, the carefully crafted schedule inked in red in my daily planner explodes in my face. A new, more binding responsibility emerges, priorities shift. Sickness pulls me from the secure shallows of my routines, and I find myself out of my depth, frantically thrashing about for solid ground.

As for the standards of health and normality themselves, these have two related qualities. First, they are typically experienced uncritically in the "natural attitude," as intrinsic preconditions of orderly social life. Second, and related to this, they show up naively or falsely as universally binding on all human beings. The adverbs "naïvely" and "falsely" are fitting, for historical and anthropological investigations demonstrate that these standards are in fact manmade and, if not entirely arbitrary, are at least highly variable. To quote Eric Cassell, they "are human inventions, . . . They have no independent existence like oak trees or snowflakes" (Cassell, 1991, 133, 105, 108).

In one culture, health may be assessed by examining a person's nose shape, breast size, or outward intelligence; in another by their pulse or temperature; in still a third by their fertility or strength. One diagnostic of male health in ancient India, still occasionally used to determine one's fitness for marriage, was the quality of the young man's *virya* = semen; a word etymologically related to the Latin *virtus*, from which we get both moral "virtue" and *virtú*—manliness and power (*Narada*, 1969 [1889], sec. 12.8–12.10). Again, while medical doctors assess the status of their patients' neurons and arteries to determine their fitness, acupuncturists attend to an entirely different system, one comprised of "meridians" or channels of *chi* (*qi*, pronounced "chee" = energy). The quality of chi in turn is said to reflect the harmony of one's yin (female) and yang (male) substances. Thus, while reflexes and blood pressure indicate organic functioning for M.D.s, traditional Chinese patients might be asked, after a thin needle is emplaced in their wrist, whether or not they feel their chi "rising."[1]

Whatever the content of the standards, relative to them are abnormalities, deviations, sicknesses: Hindu men whose semen is too watery, evil smelling, or colored; people whose nose bridges are adjudged too thick; women whose breasts are too small. Take negritude, for example, a "sickness" first identified by the father of American psychiatry and Dean of the University of Pennsylvania Medical School, Dr. Benjamin Rush, in the early 1800s (Szasz, 1970, 154–58). Its major symptom: dark skin pigmentation, a condition that Rush attributed to leprosy. To prove the connection between leprosy and negritude, Rush cited the case of a Negro slave named Henry Moss who, in the course of three years, spontaneously turned entirely white. (Today a similar condition, known as vitiligo, is observable in both black and "white" populations. About 1 percent of Americans suffer from it.) Dr. Rush argued that all the symptoms then stereotypically associated with negritude (i.e., leprosy)—wooly hair, a flat nose, thick lips, an insensitivity to hot coals and cutting (due to neuropathy), and "strong venereal desires"—could be cured by means of proper medical therapy. At the same time, he cautioned against interracial marriage on grounds that this would "tend to infect posterity" with "the disorder."

Compared to the culture of his time, Rush was a progressive thinker. He signed the Declaration of Independence, and he opposed slavery, which during the colonial era was widely thought by Christians to be a just punishment for the sins of the supposed ancestor of Africans, Ham (Gen. 9:22–25). After all, he argued, it could hardly be fair to punish a man for a disease, a condition, completely out of his control. But what needs to be emphasized here is that in posing negritude as a disease, whiteness for Rush and his colleagues was valorized. It became the standard of physical normality: "It was inconceivable to Rush that when the Negro had been cured of his affliction . . . he would have the red complexion of the American Indian or the yellow of the Asiatic" (Szasz, 1970, 158).

There exist a multitude of other, equally bizarre, examples that underscore the same point. Take "revolutiona," for example, or as it was otherwise known, "anarchia," another of Benjamin Rush's colonial-period ailments. Its defining symptom was lack of respect for the British monarch, as evidenced by a propensity to protest taxes, pen subversive screeds, or, as it was said at the time, exhibiting "an excess of the passion for liberty." After the colonies freed themselves from British rule, homegrown defenders of the New England propertied class invoked the same disorder to explain why the disenfranchised American Irish underclass continued to foment unrest. In either case, by medicalizing dissent against the reputed standards of the old order, the standards themselves were revivified and given new life. (The reader should not dismiss this as one more document of pre-scientific silliness. Consider three of today's medically recognized equivalents to anarchia: conduct disorder (CD), oppositional defiance disorder (ODD), and attention deficit hyperactivity disorder (ADHD) [Levine, 2001; Erchak and Rosenfeld, 1989].)[2]

Medical conditions that animate as much concern today as anarchia did two centuries ago are eating disorders. Again, the same sociological principle applies. In naming the different types of eating disorders—anorexia, bulimia, and obesity—something almost magical transpires. The shared prejudice that certain kinds of hunger are "sick" is objectified and the people who have these hungers are pathologized. At the same time, the standards of normal appetite are rendered into "social facts," things as concrete and substantial in their own way as mortar and bricks. Of course, unlike mortar and bricks we can't actually *see* standards of healthy appetite, any more than we can see air or gravity. But as Emile Durkheim once warned, like air and gravity, these standards can be ignored only at one's peril.

When eating disorders are publicly "awfulized" on afternoon theatres of body agony such as *Montel*, *Oprah*, or *Dr. Phil*, the standards of healthy consumption become more certain, more absolute. And when we read with pity about the victims' plights, conduct research into the causes of their conditions, and attend with relief to stories of their heroic recoveries, the standards become that much more compelling, more powerful. In this way the sick serve as our instructors. By negative example, they teach us what normality is. The sickness itself—the eating disorder, the addiction, the sexual perversion, the childhood defiance, the "leprous" black skin—are the "lesson plans."[3]

Michel Foucault writes about how asylums once served as informal tutorials for the edification of the French public (Foucault, 1965, 207–8). On Sundays, families would prepare picnic lunches, dress in their finery, and take guided tours of the facilities. There they would gape through the cell bars at the begrimed, half-naked humanity chained within. The spectacle taught witnesses an ineffaceable moral—namely, that for all of their own personal problems, at least they were not one of *them*. Sickness, then, not only helps constitute society's boundaries; it also reassures us that suspicions about our own well-being are unfounded. "I'm okay, you're okay."

It is important to remember that in speaking about the social purpose of sicknesses, we are not addressing the question of their "etiologies," their causes: the bio-psycho-social conditions independent of, prior to, and statistically associated with their appearance. That is a subject of another discussion. Our goal in this chapter is phenomenology, the depiction of the experiential parameters of health-related issues. Furthermore, we don't want to blind ourselves to the fact that however much sicknesses may help maintain social order (at least within limits) and make "normals" feel better about themselves, from the standpoint of the victims themselves they usually entail anguish and suffering.

However this may be, if it is true that sicknesses have a social purpose then it is difficult to imagine a society without them. There *must* be sicknesses, regardless of the costs accrued in trying to rid ourselves of them. As Friedrich Nietzsche once remarked apropos of enemies: sicknesses are so essential for social unity and for a personal sense of self-worth that if they didn't exist, they'd have to be invented.[4] And so they are. In 1854, when debate about the moral legitimacy of slavery was about to shatter the American republic, a peculiar epidemic was discovered flourishing amidst the African population by a prominent Louisiana physician named Samuel Cartwright: drapetomania (Gr. *drapeto* [runaway] + *mania* [mad]). It "induces the negro to run away from service," says Cartwright, "[and] is as much a disease . . . as any other species of mental alienation, and much more curable," he happily adds (Szasz, 1971). The presumed cure was to amputate the "patient's" toes.

As this vignette shows, lurking behind many ailments are "well-doers," health entrepreneurs, and medical claims-makers who market troubling concerns as medical syndromes. This being the case we can always ask, whose norms or standards of health are they? What interests do they enable? (Freund et al., 2003, 126–27). Advancing the case for negritude, drapetomania, and dysaesthesia aethiopica (still another nineteenth-century Negro disorder, the symptom of which was "paying no attention to the master's property") were well-doers concerned with keeping black people with their "stallion-like lusts" cowed and apart from the white population. In regard to ADHD and ODD, on the other hand, the advocates include drug companies looking to bolster the bottom line, pediatricians and pedagogues trying to legitimize their claims to professionalism, and worried parents seeking excuses for their child's classroom failures and delinquency.

Sickness as Deviance

To repeat, from society's standpoint sickness presents itself as a kind of deviance. It is neither a sin, nor strictly a crime. Some observers suggest that it be considered a form of passive-aggressive resistance against the standards of bodily normality and, more generally, against the routines of the ordinary life-world (Greco, 1998, 148; Freund et al., 2003, 139–41): a type of pre- or non-reflective objection. We use the prefix "non" because unlike, say, conscientious objection to war, which is carefully thought out and chosen, a sickness is rarely a matter of conscious choice. Nevertheless, by means of sickness one can communicate his or her disgust with everyday affairs. In addition to this, sickness usually provides a safe way of avoiding one's putative responsibilities as a slave, an oppressed worker, a disgruntled wife, or a bored student.

While separating them like we do here is arbitrary, we can distinguish between two basic tactics employed by disgruntled people to communicate discontent with the prevailing state of affairs. One is by directly saying "I hate this and I hate you, and I refuse to do it! So there!" The other is by "talking" with our bodies, expressing the same message through angry red faces, tears of frustration, stomachaches, fatigue, and hives; that is, by getting sick. A good example of this is *zār*.

Zār (Arabic from *ziara* = visitation) is an affliction prevalent among adult females who inhabit the highly patriarchal Muslim tribes of Sudan, Ethiopia, Somalia, and Egypt. Its symptoms include chronic pain, a lack of energy, and depression. In short, the woman doesn't quite feel like "herself." The first symptoms of *zār* typically appear around the time that a young girl reaches puberty and takes on the obligations of the veil. Like many border crossings to a new way of life, the passage into adulthood is accompanied by the shedding of blood through (painful, non-antiseptic) genital mutilation, the details of which we need not describe.[5] The condition then worsens after she marries, leaves her family, and falls under the strict supervision of a husband. It is probably not just coincidental that local folklore attributes *zār* to possession by "red spirits" of male gender. It is considered highly contagious and its incidence is said to have increased dramatically in the last few decades with the spread of Muslim fundamentalism and its insistence that married women remain cloistered behind the walls of their husbands' houses. Social anthropologists interpret *zār* as an indirect, relatively safe way of rebelling against the harsh regime under which rural Muslim women labor.

Only the intervention of other women can cure *zār*. Not surprisingly, these are women whose post-menopausal status has freed them from the veil and from the symptoms of male spirit "possession." The healing ceremony is also known as *zār*, and has been formally outlawed in Sudan since 1983. However, it continues to be celebrated, mostly underground. Conducted on Friday nights when husbands are praying at the mosque, the *zār* ritual involves the donning of a long white shirt and the offering to the spirits enticements like Coke, coffee, fruit, and perfume. The healing is viewed less as an exorcism than as a ceremonial placating of the spirit. Then, to tambourine, flute, and ululating song—each spirit is alleged to have its own preferred musical lilt—the patient is urged to dance. Usually at first she is reluctant to do so, but then she begins slowly to sway. In the end she abandons herself completely, throwing her hair back "wantonly," flailing her arms, burping, speaking boorishly. Says one participant: "the music took me over. The beat can get inside of you and make you crazy." If all goes well, the result is cathartic release from pent-up hostility (cf. Arabella, n.d.; Bizzari, n.d.).

Again, the suggestion here is that I am not just Descartes' *cogito*, a *Homo clausus*, as Monica Greco describes it (Greco, 1998, 11, 16–18, 21–22), a "true self" hiding behind my skin. Rather, I *am* this body, a body with its own wisdom (Wolf and Wolff, 1947). And often it seems to "know" more than what I can consciously admit. Just as a Freudian slip or "a friendly jest" can reveal my contempt for you, so I may be shocked, ashamed, or angered by what my body betrays about my real feelings. One such betrayal is sickness. It can be viewed as a clumsy, often misunderstood, "protolanguage" by which I convey my "dis-ease" with the world. It "somatizes" my distress over unresolved conflicts (Szasz, 1974, 107–24). Viewed in this way, disease is not so much what I *have*, but what I *do* (Becker, 2005, 83–92). It is a "surrogate truth," the proper understanding of which can, through guidance, serve as a vehicle for personal liberation from a hitherto unresolved life dilemma.

In their *Studies in Hysteria*, Sigmund Freud and Joseph Breuer tell the story of Anna O (Freud and Breuer, 1952, 22–23). Anna O's father, whom she deeply loved, fell ill of pneumonia. He lingered on the edge of death for months, only to eventually succumb. For the first few weeks, Anna devoted her entire waking life to his care, until in time "to no one's surprise," her own health began to deteriorate. She lost her appetite, weakened, and became so anemic that, "to her great sorrow" she was no longer "allowed to continue nursing the patient." Even under a doctor's care, however, her condition did not improve. Instead, after her father died she developed a lingering cough, chronic headaches, vertigo, and severe muscle tension in her upper back, neck, and arms.

Thomas Szasz suggests that Anna O was essentially an oppressed, unpaid sick-nurse, coerced into the role by her father's helplessness and her own relationship to him. Middle-class women in Anna O's day were expected to care for their sick fathers; a nanny watched over the children. Hiring a professional servant would have created a moral conflict because it would be taken as proof that she didn't really love her father after all. The progression of symptoms after she was relieved of her duties can be understood as a somatizing of the guilt she felt over having that suspicion confirmed. In any case, according to Szasz, Anna O's situation is exactly the reverse of the modern mother who is trapped by her small children and sees her parents' care farmed out to experts. The health consequences for both, he concludes, are identical.

The state of having no words for one's feelings is technically known as alexithymia (Greek *a* [lack] + *lexis* [word] + *thymos* [emotion]) (Sifneos, 1973; Sifneos, 1996; Greco, 1998, 131–58).[6] Alexithymia should not be considered a cause of any particular disease—that is, a condition that is either necessary or sufficient for a physical affliction to occur. At most it should be viewed a contributory "risk factor" in the development of a disease, and/or as a psychological state that can frustrate attempts at alleviating one (Greco, 1998, 146).

With no pretense at being exhaustive, we can list the kinds of people who, unable to articulate what Greco calls "forbidden truths," communicate their distress either through a bona fide organic disease, through a self-destructive compulsion, or by means of a chronic "somatoform" condition like fibromyalgia. First, are those rendered mute by the very violence of their traumas: rape victims, benumbed war casualties, refugees from tsunamis or earthquakes. Then there are those who are silent because they simply lack words to frame their plight, as indicated by their flat, boring, distractive responses to queries about how they are feeling: "I can't say," "I don't know," or, most pointedly, "nothing." These types have been described by psychotherapists as human "shells without cores" (Greco, 1998, 136). There are also those for whom the use of rebellious words is tabooed (e.g., children denied the right to their native tongue in schools). Then, there are those who are not explicitly forbidden to speak, and are linguistically equipped to do so, but who are overly shy or polite: "What would people think?" "I don't want to hurt anybody's feelings." In the literature, these are sometimes labeled "normopaths," outwardly well-adjusted, but inwardly unhappy people (138).

We can add to this list, conspirators of silence: two or more people who share an interest in not airing their dirty laundry in public, such as members of incestuous families, alcoholic enablers, and closeted gays. There are "codes of silent omission," as Eviatar Zerubavel calls them, the practice of using misleading euphemisms to hide an otherwise unseemly truth about the world. Finally, there is "meta-silence" wherein co-conspirators deny the fact of their self-imposed silence, studiously ignoring the elephant in the room (Zerubavel, 2006, 52–63). Whatever the reason, "the day we see the truth and [don't] . . . speak it is the day we begin to die" (86). Or, more accurately, we begin to sicken.

The reasons for this are not hard to discern. Verbal inhibition involves emotional labor (Hochschild, 1983, 35–55). Whether this is "shallow" (in the sense of controlling one's outward gestures while keeping their inner feelings intact) or "deep" (altering the feelings themselves), emotional work entails immediate physiological costs. When these are cumulative, they may be physically compromising. Hans Selye, the world's foremost expert on the subject, has itemized some of the characteristic "diseases of adaptation" to chronic stress: elevated cholesterol, high blood pressure, susceptibility to viral infections, sleeping disorders, ulcers, autoimmune diseases, and possibly cancer (Selye, 1976). On the other hand, research suggests that there are definite health benefits that follow from writing or just talking about the death of one's spouse, their own homosexual desires, or their holocaust traumas (Pennebaker, 1997, 202–25, 30–35, 84–86, 216–18). These include increased immune T-cell function (35–37), lower blood pressure (48–52), and increased congruency of hemispheric brain waves (52–55). Evidently, these payoffs are not a product of emotional catharsis as such, ala *zār* healing. Rather, they are contingent to the sense of empowerment enjoyed when one externalizes a challenging situation and "downloads" it onto paper (96–98).[7]

This may be the basis of the otherwise inexplicable "spontaneous healings" reported to occur in support groups where participants who share a disorder learn to put their rage into poetry and essays, and to acknowledge their complicity in their own suffering. This is true not just for cardiac surgery patients, AIDS victims, and cancer sufferers (Rijke, 1985), but also addicts, cripples, and women in abusive relations. Significantly, it is not uncommon for such groups to organize into political lobbies to change prevailing standards of normality. The most notable recent example of this is passage of the Americans with Disabilities Act in 1990. The ADA, of course, does not rid victims of their impairments, but it does force institutions receiving federal funds to rearrange space, patterns of movement, and services to accommodate them. This effectively normalizes what had previously been beyond the pale. Those once stigmatized as death carriers and exiled from decent company are now being mainstreamed into the ordinary lifeworld as "people just like us." Naturally, there remains a good bit of resistance to assimilation on the part of self-proclaimed proponents of "traditional values." Witness the furious fight against decriminalizing sodomy laws and for outlawing gay marriage. But if recent history is a basis for prediction, inclusiveness is probably inevitable. As proof, look at what happened to the "disease" of negritude.

Deviance as Sickness

All social deviation disrupts the world. Its variations prefigure chaos and, ultimately, death. But exactly *how* deviation discloses itself and how it is handled changes over time. This is because in every advanced society there is a struggle between three elites over jurisdiction of stubborn bodies: religious authorities, legal authorities, and medical authorities. As different elites achieve ascendancy, the ways that deviance is experienced change, sometimes dramatically.

To be sure, this is to pose the situation a little too simplistically. As we shall see below, there is considerable overlap in how priests, clerks, and doctors frame deviance. It is also true that whenever a single church monopolizes the means of psychical coercion over a territory, as Roman Catholicism did during the European Middle Ages, clergy often serve *as* government officials. (Indeed, the word "clerk" comes from the word "cleric.") Furthermore, religious leaders and their argot are frequently used to accomplish quasi-medical purposes (or vice versa). One example of this is Alcoholics Anonymous (AA), whose twelve-step program serves as the template for treating a wide variety of addictions, from shopping and drugs to sex.

Just months after the prohibition amendment to the Constitution was repealed in 1933, effectively decriminalizing alcohol consumption, the American Medical Association voted to recognize alcoholics as "valid patients" (Szasz, 1975, 2–17, 177–84). With this declaration, responsibility for dealing with alcoholism was formally transferred out of the hands of the police into those of doctors. But these were not doctors of the sort familiar to us today, proponents of secular science. The two founders of AA, Bill Wilson and "Dr. Bob," were instead evangelical Christians.

Their *Big Book* details how the original twelve-step program was expressly modeled after the prototypical Midwestern Methodist revival meetings of their youth (Alcoholics Anonymous, 2002). First is the examination of conscience during which the alcoholic is required to undertake a "moral inventory." This is followed by confession of their "sickness" (read: sin) to the assembly of fellow inebriates. Then comes redemptive surrender to (originally in Methodism, the saving grace of) an unnamed "higher power," after which the born-again addict pays "restitution" (does penance) to those s/he has harmed. In sum, the founding of AA offers a classic instance of decriminalization, followed by medicalization, which on closer view is actually a remoralizing of one form of waywardness.

The history of psychiatry is replete with examples of physicians who end up serving as non-uniformed law enforcement officers (Szasz, 1965). When psychiatry originated during what Foucault calls "The Great Confinement" (ca. 1800), an event we will return to momentarily, it was given responsibility to monitor the mental health of populations (Foucault, 1965, 38–64). It accomplished this by devising tests that could separate raving maniacs (who would be cared for in asylums) from malingerers and cowards, who would be punished in prison. This task was later expanded to include the determination of criminal defendants to stand trial, to aid in sentencing, and of providing assistance to law enforcement agencies in dealing with domestic enemies. Under Communist rule, psychiatrists were enlisted to help quell political dissent. In the "workers' paradise" of Yugoslavia during the 1950s, for example, then–vice president Milovan Djilas was imprisoned in a hospital for the criminally insane after he was diagnosed as suffering from "hallucinations." It seems he was seeing social classes in the very place where Marxist theory says there can be none. As if this were not bad enough, while undergoing group therapy, he failed to exhibit "insight into his condition," insisting that he was perfectly fine. This, naturally, led to his being subjected to a more painful, humiliating "treatment plan."[8]

But let us ignore these fascinating subtleties for the moment and focus on the proposition being entertained here. At an accelerating pace since the dawn of the modern era (ca. 1600) priestly authority has been taken over by police, whose role is now in the process of being usurped by physicians.[9] As a result, the nature of deviance has changed. These alterations can be summarized by the phrase "medicalization of deviance." It is reflected in four developments.

First and most tellingly, the same general sorts of deviance have evolved from sins into crimes and from crimes into sicknesses (see table 4.1). One document of this is the explosion of mental and behavioral syndromes after 1950, at the very moment that the rhetoric of sin was disappearing from everyday Euro-American discourse. "Whatever became of sin?" Karl Menninger asked in 1973 (Menninger, 1973). If he were alive today, Menninger might take comfort to learn of efforts to reverse the situation, including in his hometown of Topeka, Kansas. With the financial support of federal grant monies, Christian fundamentalists have recently mounted fierce campaigns to reposition themselves as arbiters of body matters in place of "secular progressive" doctors (like Menninger himself), particularly regarding substance abuse issues and problematic sexuality. Resurrecting the neo-Calvinist dogma of mankind's inherent depravity, they have even put up resistance to vaccination programs intended to avert the spread of human papillomavirus (HPV) and with it, of genital warts and cervical cancer. The fear is that vaccination might encourage adolescent debauchery (Goldberg, 2007, 106–33).

Table 4.1.   Sins and Selected Corresponding Modern Sicknesses

The Seven Deadly Sins	Seven Corresponding Sickness
Vanity (*superbia*)	Narcissistic Personality Disorder (NPD)
Envy (*invidia*)	Social Anxiety Disorder (SAD)
Anger (*ira*)	Intermittent Explosive Disorder (IED)
Gluttony (*gula*)	Substance Use Disorder (SUD)
Greed (*avaritia*)	Obsessive Compulsive Disorder (OCD)
Lust (*luxuria*)	Sexual Addiction Disorder (SAD)
Lethargy (*acedia*)	Depressive Disorder (DD)

Second, the presumed cause of deviance has shifted. Sin is explained by an absence of moral virtue, an inability to control one's sinful proclivities. Crime, in contrast, is identified by a particular kind of *presence*, specifically, as it is known in law, *mens rea*, a conscious intention to do wrong. Without proof of *mens rea*, defendants are judged innocent, perhaps because their youth renders them incapable of forming criminal intent. A sickness, on the hand, is an altogether different matter. It is not a choice made by an active agent. Rather, it is a tragedy that befalls a passive victim. Thus, while sins like sodomy and gluttony, for example, speak to a lack of strength to resist the kinds of temptations faced by *all* human beings, the comparable medical conditions of homosexuality and alcoholism are said to be *impulses* that healthy individuals do not have. They are caused by forces outside the victim's control—in the case of homosexuality, by a "gay" gene, or, in regard to alcoholism, by a gene that marks them as a so-called gamma. This is a person who is said to be "allergic" to alcohol, and is thus prone to addiction. The gay or gamma genes become inheritable conditions that can only be suffered, or, possibly in the future, cured by gene-splicing, but certainly not to be condemned.

Third, the remedies for deviance have mutated. Sins call for confession to a priest who then recommends penance; felonies are remediated by punishment. Sicknesses, on the other hand, require medical intervention. All of these can be, and usually are, painful. ("Penance" and "punishment" both come from the Latin word for pain [*poena*].) However, the understanding of the pain differs in each case. The purpose of penance is purificatory atonement, the re-establishment of the believer's "at-one-ment" with God, a psychic state designated by the term "grace." Grace readies the believer to accept God's miraculous saving power. The pains of criminal justice have a different meaning. Their object is not to save souls, but to rebalance the felon's debts to society. Lastly, medical cures are undertaken for the patient's health, their physical and emotional well-being in *this* world, not their salvation in the next.

Fourth, the technologies of interrogation and the administration of pain have changed. They have moved from the confessional booth and inquisitional tribunal of the church, through the police grilling, trial proceeding, and prison cell, to the clinical dossier, hospital room, and surgical suite.

As indicated above, this picture is overly simplistic. In the first place, although it is true that atonement, justice, and health are variant enterprises, each with their own incantations, equipment, and accommodations, the three words echo off each other. Health suggests wholeness, which speaks to at-one-ment, the latter of which implies non-dividedness and harmony. But harmony calls out the idea of balance and therefore of justice.

The word "sickness" has comparable resonances. To be sick is to ail, to be not well. Unwell is an adverbial form of the noun phrase "not good." But to be "not good" is tantamount to being bad which, at least in extreme cases, is evil. The Latin term for evil is *crimen*. In sum, then, while sin, crime, and sickness are distinguishable, they are far from separable.

Michel Foucault traces the medicalization of deviance to an event he calls the Great Confinement, and to the rise of a uniquely modern institution: the medical clinic (Foucault, 1975). According to Foucault the first European hospitals were church-run refuges for the feeding, sheltering, and clothing—i.e., the hospitality—of the "polymorphous poor": vagrants, the elderly, orphans, and the mad. Under the rationalizing impulse of the French Revolution, fearing that the "pestilential domain" of this kind of hospital was a threat to national well-being, each type of "unreason" (i.e., deviance) began to be parceled out from the others and confined to its own facility: lunatics to the asylum, criminals to prison, "worthy paupers" to the poorhouse, and the sick to clinics. There, each would be subjected to the "gaze" of their own cadre of trained specialists. Those who resisted help were considered "guilty of ingratitude" to society for the care they received (84). Foucault goes on to say that it was in the madhouse, prison, workhouse, and clinic that the empirical sciences, respectively, of psychiatry, penology, welfare, and, most importantly for our purposes, biomedicine, emerged; each science charged with the responsibility to "produce docile bodies." It was at this point that disease in the sense that we are using the term in this book, an observable organic pathology, assumed ontological status as an object separate from sin, insanity, crime, and home-lessness, and physicians began their vocational ascent in the so-cial hierarchy. The results became immediately evident, particularly in regard to the management of bodily orifices.[10]

Ladies' Conditions

In Western civilization female flesh has been a perennial object of suspicion by males who have comprised the vast majority of philosophers, lawyers, doctors, and theologians (Schott, 1988; Lederer, 1968). Especially problematic is the supposed core of fe-male essence: the uterus. Being the doorway both of life and, through menstrual blood and the threat it poses to male virility, of death, the uterus has always evoked a combination of fasci-nation and horror.

In Christian tradition female genital phobia was framed in the language of sin. The reader should already be familiar with the refrain: she is the Devil's gateway; the deceiver, Satan's con-sort; cause of mankind's Fall. In the *Malleus Malificarum* ("Ham-mer of Witches"), a notorious inquisitional guidebook from the fifteenth century, the Dominican authors account for the sup-posed female propensity to witchery by citing the insatiable ap-petite of a womb "that can never say 'enough'" (a gloss on Prov. 30:16; Sprenger and Krämer, 1970 [1486], 47).

Except for pockets of fundamentalist reaction, commentary like this today is largely dismissed as archaic. For ours is a pro-gressive age, one in which the beguiling terror of female flesh has transmogrified. Just as African slaves in the nineteenth cen-tury advanced from being perpetrators of evil into carriers of disease (leprosy), fear of female flesh has become medicalized. In enlightened circles, she is seen less as a stumbling block to sal-vation than as a victim of one or more "ladies' conditions," syn-dromes that require professional medical attention.[11] Barbara Ehrenreich and Deirdre English (2005) provide an account of one step in this development.

Following the Civil War (ca. 1865), informed American publics began noticing a peculiar malady within the female

WASP population, the symptoms of which were remarkably like those of *zār*. And like *zār*, they commenced around the time of puberty, only to increase in severity after courtship and marriage: headaches, pelvic distress, digestive problems, faintness, fatigue, choking sensations, difficulty in breathing, etc.; "a terrible decay of female health across the nation," lamented one physician.

The ailment attracted the attention of period gynecologists, most notably Dr. S. Weir Mitchell, then Philadelphia's preeminent female specialist. They made the following "discovery": female functions are inherently pathological. This appeared to explain why the more "feminine" (read: white, prosperous, and genteel) she was, the more susceptible she seemed to invalidism; and vice versa, why swarthy, "unladylike" immigrant women from eastern Europe, who were then flooding America's shores, did not share the debilitation. Said one doctor, "thus women are treated for diseases of the stomach, liver, kidneys, heart, lungs, etc. . . . But [the distresses are] sympathetic reactions or symptoms of one disease, namely, a disease of the womb" (Ehrenreich and English, 2005, 134). The poor ladies were victims of hysteria (Gr. *hystera* = uterus). They suffer from unfulfilled wombs! "Many a young [woman] is battered and forever crippled on the breakers of puberty," opined Dr. Engleman, in 1900 president of the American Gynecological Society.

> If [she] crosses these unharmed and is not dashed to pieces on the rock of childbirth, [she] may still ground on the ever-recurring shallows of menstruation, and lastly upon the final bar of menopause, ere protection is found in the unruffled waters of the harbor beyond the reach of sexual storms (121).

For centuries, Catholic priests had resisted attempts by secular physicians to gain a foothold in the territory of the female body over which the church had long enjoyed exclusive control. In spite of this, by 1650 the tics, insomnias, anorexia, hair pulling, gnashing of teeth, and hiccups reported by women were beginning to find a place in medical nosology (Gilman et al., 1993, 114–16).[12] What clerics had earlier seen as "stigmata" of sorcery, of "wicked wombs" being diabolically "possessed" by Satan, doctors were coming to redefine as "symptoms" of "disease," conditions entirely explicable in naturalistic terms. And what had earlier been characterized as heresy and dealt with through exorcism, torture, and murder, physicians began to treat rationally and humanely by medicine and machines.

The church condemned efforts by doctors to demystify female complaints, accusing them of perpetrating an even more egregious abomination, "notorious heresy." *Haeresis est maxima opera maleficarum non credere*, screamed the *Malleus Malificarum*: "To disbelieve in witchcraft is the greatest of heresies" (Sprenger and Krämer, 1970 [1486], 8–9, 56). Dr. Edward Jorden, one of the accused, replied by ridiculing the "supernaturalists" with their "popishe impostures."

> Another signe of a supernaturall power they make to be due & orderly returning of the fits, when they keepe their just day and houre, which we call periods. . . . This accident is common to diverse other chronicall diseases, as headaches, gowtes, Epilepsies, Tertians, Quartans & c. so it is often observed in [hysteria] as is sufficiently proved. . . . Another argument of theirs is the offense in eating, or drinking, as if the Divell ment to choake them therewith. But this symptom is also ordinaire in uterin affects. (Gilman et al., 1993, 122)

When investigations of corpses in the newly erected clinics of the nineteenth century disproved the ancient Greek theory of the wandering womb—that unfulfilled *hystera* literally migrate to different body sites causing convulsions, paralyses, and pain (Lefkowitz, 1996)—a more empirically plausible theory was devised. The womb still suffers, it was agreed, but it remains permanently affixed to the abdomen by ligaments. Thus it is not the womb itself that roves nomadically through the body in search of fulfillment; it is the foul vapors of unrequited love; it is congested uterine blood; or it is nerve impulses radiating outward from the distressed organ. These vapors, humors, or discharges eventually insinuate themselves into porous body parts of the victim, occasioning her "wombiness." Due to her delicacy, "frail nerves," and sympathetic habits, in other words, the woman "encloses a perpetual possibility of hysteria" (Foucault, 1965, 154). Her very femininity, openness, and sensitivity render her susceptible to illness: "Terrible state! . . . This is the torment of effeminate souls" (157).

The recommended palliatives for hysteria reflected the primitive level of medical knowledge then prevalent (Ehrenreich and English, 2005, 135–37, 144–47). Routine cases called for bed rest and the avoidance of unpleasant sensations, including the husband's bad breath. This could be supplemented with a prescription of iron filings to increase her "density" or solidity, and make her less susceptible to sympathetic impulses. Then there was the application of leeches to the vagina to relieve congestion, injections into it of soporifics, such as warm linseed oil or liquid marshmallow, or the placement therein of animal excrement suppositories. The latter practice has since been assimilated into modern medicine in the form of estrogen replacement therapy, which uses concentrated pregnant mare urine. If all else failed, doctors were told that "a single string still vibrates in them, that of pain; have courage to pluck it" (Foucault, 1965, 182). That is, deal with the offending part surgically, by hysterectomy: removing the uterus altogether.

For the Greeks, the unfulfilled womb was said to wander in search of a child. By the late nineteenth century, its hunger was increasingly being reinscribed in sexual terms. Sexual gratification was seen as a cure for hysteria, with marriage its guarantor (Gilman et al., 1993, 135). For widows and spinsters, alternatives were proposed. One was pelvic massage to "hysterical paroxysm," preferably done by a female *obstetrix*. Given that this could take hours, in 1873 the first electricity-driven vibrators were introduced, ten years before the iron or the vacuum cleaner. Sears and Roebuck would later market these devices as household appliances (Maines, 1999).

It isn't necessary to detail Ehrenreich's and English's sociological explanation for the epidemic of hysteria in the nineteenth century, except to say that it reminds us of that posited above for *zār*. Carefree Victorian girls were being thrust into a life of enclosed idleness, relegated to being ornaments for ostentatious display by their husbands at the public garden, theater, salon, assembly, or church. To accomplish her purpose of impression management, it was incumbent on the wife to orchestrate gesture, gait, verbal affect, and dress just so, being at once flirtatiously coy yet coldly disciplined: smiling, blinking, blushing, weeping, and swooning in calibrated ways and at precise moments. "Forever balancing over the abyss" of impropriety and scandal, many wives "buckled" under the pressure (Gilman et al., 1993, 160–65). They began to somatize their distress in conventionally acceptable ways— namely, by coming down with the "vapors," becoming sickly.

As the twentieth century progressed hysteria largely disappeared from medical discourse (Micale, 1993). Recently, however, reports of new disorders have surfaced, with comparable symptoms. One is multiple personality disorder (MPD); another is depression (Hirshbein, 2006).[13] It is not necessary for us to determine which claim, if either, is true. What is important to keep in mind is that female flesh remains an object of suspicion.

By 1900 Phillippe Pinel, Jean-Martin Charcot, and Jean Esquirol, the luminaries of French psychiatry, had already destroyed the plausibility of the theological account for female afflictions (Szasz, 1970, 68–81). What began in 1650 as a hypothesis tentatively entertained had by now become medical dogma. She is not a heretic, the doctors agreed, but a hysteric. For all this, however, Woman was still subject to the gaze of male authority, and her fleshly essence alleged to be the source of her suffering. Freed by secular progressive thinkers from the libel of being allied with the Antichrist, she now assumed the status of patient, congenitally bound to Unreason.

Notes

1. Robert O. Becker, a celebrated researcher in electro-medicine and co-author of *The Body Electric*, once conducted federally funded research on chi. He reportedly found that the electrical current running along the so-called H meridian is stronger than that in nearby nerves (Reichmanis et al., 1979).

2. There is an immense, rapidly growing literature on the "social construction," as it is phrased, of issues of public concern, including missing children, rock and rap music, drunk driving, immigration and terrorism, the AIDS epidemic, infertility, and the crack attack, as well as spousal and elder abuse. Some of these concerns, with the help of allied health professionals and pharmaceutical manufacturers, have been turned into sicknesses. For an introduction to the invention of social problems, see Best (1989) and Best (1995).

3. Child abuse was first identified as a medical condition in 1962 in *The Journal of the American Medical Association* (*JAMA*) (Johnson, 1989, 6). The report and accompanying editorial condemn child-rearing practices that only a few years earlier had been widely used by parents to instill discipline, and which find support in Old Testament teachings. By medically pathologizing traditional Judeo-Christian child-rearing techniques, *JAMA* implicitly endorsed a kinder, gentler way of compelling obedience, one more congenial to the sensibilities of an affluent, secular, suburban American population.

4. "Imagine 'the enemy' as conceived by the man [who would reform the world] and here precisely is his deed, his creation: he has conceived the 'evil enemy,' 'the evil one'—and indeed as the fundamental basis from which he then derives as an afterimage and counter-instance, a 'good one'—himself" (Nietzsche, 1969, part 1, sec. 10).

5. Interested readers may consult Boddy (1989, 49–51, 57–60).

6. See also Lumley et al. (1996), Taylor (1984), and Taylor (1991).

7. There remain serious questions of adequate design controls in much of this research. Even advocates of talking things into clarity admit that it doesn't work for everyone, and many don't appear to need it (Pennebaker, 1997, 87–88).

8. A similar case concerns world-renowned American poet, Ezra Pound. After World War II, he was arrested for his fascist radio speeches that had been aired from Italy. For his insistence that his broadcasts were not treasonous, plus his "abnormally grandiose" style and verbosity, Pound was adjudged "incurably insane," and spent thirteen years undergoing "treatment" at St. Elizabeth's hospital in Washington D.C. (Szasz, 1970, 29, 315).

9. The Quaker-inspired penitentiary, first established in Pennsylvania in 1829, offers a unique example of how penance and punishment can be conflated in practice. It constitutes a notable exception to our proposition. Here, instead of inflicting pain on prisoners, as was the traditional practice at the New York state prison, the idea was to allow convicts to reform themselves by placing them in solitary confinement. This presumably gave them the opportunity to undertake examinations of conscience and be rehabilitated.

10. In 1862 sodomy, a so-called criminal sin, punishable in principle by death in colonial Massachusetts, was reframed into a psychopathology, becoming a "perversion" known as "homosexuality." "Heterosexuality," the considered medical standard of normality, would not be coined until several years later (Katz, 1995, 20–22, 51–54). At the same time onanism, named after the biblical character Onan, who was punished with death by Yahweh for having "spilt his seed on the ground" to avoid impregnating his deceased brother's wife (Gen. 38:9–10), evolved into "masturbatory psychosis." Although the term "masturbation" (from Latin *manu* [manual] + *stupration* [defilement]) had been coined several decades earlier during the revolutionary period, its identification as a disease was new. Clinically, the symptoms of masturbatory psychosis included nearsightedness, split hair ends, indolence, pimples, and sheepishness. It was said to be responsible for male impotence, epilepsy, and *tabes*

dorsalis (body-wasting); and in women, for uterine hemorrhage, leucorrhea (vaginal discharge), and cancer. Physicians proposed many remedies for this terrifying condition, including spiked male chastity belts and cauterization of the clitoris with white-hot instruments (Szasz, 1970, 180–206).

11. There is an immense literature on the medicalization of female flesh, some of it picturing it as part of a techno-patriarchal conspiracy (cf. Corea, 1986). This is not our position.

Examples of medicalization include premenstrual discomfort, which is now late luteal phase distrophic disorder (LLPDD) (Bell, 1990) and infertility, a "disease" calling for ART (assisted reproductive technologies). Included among the latter are GIFT (gamete intra-fallopian transfer) and BABI (blastomere analysis before implantation) (Davis-Floyd and Dumit, 1998). Failure to experience orgasm, once a sign of feminine virtue, is now a medical condition known as female sexual dysfunction disorder (FSDD). It is treated by an armory of mechanical devices and pills (Maines, 1999). The otherwise natural state of menopause is now written of as estrogen depletion disease (EDD), "a deficiency disease . . . similar to diabetes. . . . A horror of living decay" (Wilson, 1968). Birthing finds itself supervised by doctors for whom it is increasingly a surgical procedure (Banks, 1999). In America, close to one-fourth of all births are Caesarian sections. The number is 20 percent in England.

12. Although this may be due to a mistranslation of Hippocrates' aphorisms by nineteenth-century physicians, the claim was made that hysteria was recognized in ancient Greek medicine, if not earlier (Gilman et al., 1993, 8).

13. MPD was first formally acknowledged as a bona fide disease by the American Psychiatric Association in 1980 in the *Diagnostic and Statistical Manual* (*DSM-III*) (Acocella, 1998). Soon afterward what had earlier been a notably rare condition grew to epidemic proportions. During the decade after 1985 more than forty thousand MPD diagnoses were confirmed. Critics believe that part of this was due to the fact of celebrities like Roseanne Barr, LaToya Jackson, and Oprah Winfrey airing accounts of MPD on afternoon talk shows. Roseanne once claimed to have been inhabited by over twenty different personalities, including Piggy, Bambi, and Fucker (68).

5

The Diseases of Medicine

Physical and mental troubles show up in society as sicknesses—deviations to be corrected. To patients, they disclose themselves as illnesses. To doctors, ailments present themselves as diseases to be cured. True, none of these—sickness, illness, or disease—is entirely separate from the others. Yet it is important for us not to obscure their differences. As Edmund Husserl might have expressed it, sickness, illness, and disease each have their own "eidetic [ideal] essence," their structural qualities without which they could not be the things they are (Husserl, 1977, 69–72).[1] This chapter is concerned exclusively with the ideal essence, so to say, of disease. It is a concept best understood in the context of a more encompassing account of the *Körper*.

Körper

The basic unit of analysis in biomedicine is the *Körper*, a system of chemical (hormonal), electrical (neurological), and mechanical (skeletal) functions. In medical science the corporeal body is both decontextualized (removed from its social-cultural milieu) and de-animated (divested of any semblance of spirit or soul-stuff). In other words, it is depersonalized. Medical science does not treat persons as such; it deals with human organisms.

The medical profession is perfectly aware of its own deper-
sonalizing trajectory, and medical schools everywhere are ac-
tively trying to rectify it. However, students report that their
classmates often complain bitterly that courses intended to help
them relate more personally with patients interfere with study
time (Oransky and Savitz, 1998). Ivan Oransky and Sean Savitz,
two prominent physicians who were still attending America's
leading medical colleges when they issued their report, claim that
a paucity of social skills is already evident among first-year medical students, whose emotional maturity lags far behind that of
their age peers. They account for this by noting that their entire
lives up to that point have involved getting good grades. Among
other things, this has meant avoiding out-of-class relationships
and shunning undergraduate humanities and arts courses that
might have broadened their perspectives. Once in medical school
the pattern continues, say Oransky and Savitz. Students are
awarded honors and prizes on the basis of exam scores, not for
their interpersonal skills or practical life experiences, and certainly not for subjective considerations like bedside manner. And
this does not end after graduation. The typical postgraduate resi-
dent undergoes an almost inhuman grind for two years, with
work "days" sometimes lasting thirty-six hours. Although the os-
tensible goal of this procedure is to train young doctors to effectively manage time, the result is that they often come to dread
their patients, if not to despise them altogether. David Shlim confesses that he once hoped that a middle-aged woman wheeled
into the emergency room at the hospital of his residency would
die so that he could get back to sleep (Shlim and Chokyi, 2006, 1).[2]

Findings from recent experiments suggest that Shlim's response may be far from unique. After witnessing acupuncture
needles being placed in the hands, feet, and mouths of patients,
magnetic resonance imagery (MRIs) showed that different centers in the brains of lay people were aroused than in those of
medical experts. Lay viewers displayed activation of regions associated with pain processing and, at least according to researchers, sympathy. In contrast, the brains of the medical
professionals lit up in areas associated with emotional control
and rational thought (Cheng et al., 2007).

According to Oransky and Savitz, student doctors display little sympathy for their patients because they have neither the hours nor the energy to do so. But there is another, more straightforward, explanation for the observation. It is, simply, that sympathy has little, if any, legitimate place in biomedicine. This is because biomedicine is, for better or worse, a science and the conclusions of science are to be based on "empirical vigilance receptive only to the evidence of [the] visible" (Foucault, 1975, xiii), on what can be seen by independent, emotionally detached investigators. But this implies that biomedicine, at least ideally, must overlook the inwardness of living; that the subjective dimension of personhood be ignored (Greco, 1998, 71).[3]

The history of modern medicine is a centuries-long narrative of how oral accounts of patients' "lack of ease" have been superseded by technically mediated "discourses on tissues" (to quote Foucault). One pivotal moment in this history concerns the invention of the stethoscope by René Laennec in 1819.

The stethoscope enabled physicians to directly attend to ("auscultate") the poundings and rumblings of the heart and lungs. The price for this, however, was that the patient's voice first had to be silenced lest it interfere with an accurate sounding. The diagnostic advantages conferred by repressing the patient's words soon led to the introduction of other observational tools: the ophthalmoscope, for example, for peering into the eye; the rhinoscope, the nose; the otoscope, the ear; the gastroscope, the stomach. With each innovation, the focus of medicine was deflected further and further away from the actual lived concerns of patients toward the objective metrics of instrumentality.

Handheld scopes eventually led to the X-ray, which was discovered largely by accident in 1895 by nuclear chemist Wilhelm Roentgen. X-rays allowed physicians to penetrate the opaque shield of the patient's skin altogether and gaze directly at what were originally foggy simulacra of their organs (Svenaeus, 2000, 30–31). This in turn gave way in the 1980s to computerized axial tomography (the CAT scan), which produces high-resolution photographs of one millimeter cross-sections of these same organs. A decade later, the MRI (magnetic resonance imagery) took this one step further, yielding three-dimensional pictures of organs in "real time." This permitted an even more detailed and intimate view of our flesh.

Both MRI and CAT scan technologies are based on the assumption that the body is in reality little more than a composite of atomic particles, susceptible to the influence of radio waves. It would be hard to exaggerate the significance of this assumption. First, it lends support to the proposition, originally entertained by René Descartes, that the body is in essence an organization of minute, motile particles. Second, and more pointedly for our purposes, it highlights Hans Jonas's claim that what he calls an "ideology of death" has come to prevail, among other places in the modern world, in the very heart of medical science itself.

The Cosmology of Death

In *The Phenomenon of Life* (1966), Jonas relates the story of how, during our era, the once-dominant ontology of the premodern world—vitalism—was overthrown. Vitalism or animism is the conviction that the entire cosmos is alive; not just trees and beasts, but fire, water, storms, and stone (cf. Chesterton, 1959 [1908]). In this worldview, death obtrudes as an incongruity, an oddity, an anomaly in need of an explanation. In the ancient world, such explanations typically took the form of death denials. However much they differ, Jonas argues, all major world religions saw death as a mere appearance, not as an actuality. It is a stage in the transmutation of what *truly* is into another, higher level, of existence. Death means liberation from the physical constraints of the body-grave and its assorted attachments.

At the outset of the modern era (ca. 1600 CE) the fundamental terms of metaphysical discourse began to shift dramatically, says Jonas. An ontology of matter emerged. The world came to be conceived as a material field comprised of inanimate objects moved by laws of inertia and motion. Vitalistic thinking was expunged. The attribution of psychic powers to plants, stones, and water was ridiculed as "anthropomorphism," the projection of human qualities onto matter. Descartes, one of the chief spokesmen for this development, condemned anthropomorphism as "scientific treason," calling it a "defilement of philosophy." In place of a teleology of ultimate ends, the movements of bodies would be attributed by Cartesians to the "ergs" of physical science.[4] The premodern enchanted garden disappeared. What remained was a residue of material stuff, things with extension, measurable, and subject to natural laws formulated in algebraic terms. In this new way of seeing, *death* now became the ontological essence of beings, life the exception. And just as death earlier was accounted for by viewing it as a variation of life, now life came to be understood in terms of the corpse: "To reduce life to . . . lifeless[ness] is . . . precisely the task set to modern biological science by the goal of 'science' as such" (Jonas, 1966, 11). But now, Jonas continues, a troubling problem arose, namely, that "when it [i.e., life] really becomes the same with the sameness of its material contents . . . it ceases to live" (75–76). In other words, life as a vital force becomes an "egregious misfit" (Zaner, 1981, 14), an inexplicable "ontological surprise" (Jonas, 1966, 79).[5]

At first, the effort to replace animate life with lifeless stuff was restricted to the realm of non-human creatures, to "automata," as Descartes called them: cats, dogs, and birds. Human beings, who alone possessed minds or souls, maintained their difference as free, purposive agents. Soon enough, however, this "fragile division" collapsed; the scientific gaze was turned back on humanity itself (Evernden, 1992, 88–96). Mankind now became automatized. "Soul" was rendered into a word whose use indicated sloppy thinking; consciousness was spoken of as an epiphenomenon; mind-stuff was reduced to brain function.

The first written expression of this doctrine is attributable to the French physician Julien Offray de La Mettrie (1709–1751) in his *L'homme machine*, "Machine Man."[6] Here, La Mettrie ridicules Descartes, along with a handful of other "idle theorists," for the "mistake," as he calls it, of giving man two substances—mind and body—when the witness of our own eyes, he says, proves there is but one: mindless matter.

These words were considered such an affront to human dignity at the time that La Mettrie's text, along with his effigy, was burned in public. In the following decades, resistance to his ideas would be mounted both by Christian moralists and by secular romantics, such as German life-philosopher Wilhelm Dilthey and his French counterpart, Henri Bergson.[7] In the halls of academic science, however, the objections became progressively muted. Eventually they were silenced altogether. Today, in experimental psychology, thinking is operationally defined as a series of electrochemical synapses traceable on the readout of an electroencephalogram (EEG). It is increasingly common to hear that, strictly speaking, humans do not really "act" at all. Rather, like La Mettrie's machines, they "operate" according to their internal chemistries and/or the "reinforcement schedules" that condition them (cf. Skinner, 1971).

As we noted in the last chapter, the institutional setting for the emergence of an empirically based mechanical medicine was the late eighteenth-century French teaching hospital. It was here that *Körper* first found itself elevated in stature to the ground of knowledge for positive medicine. In its investigation the mysteries of human life were presumed to be made intelligible. The lived-body (*Leib*) was left to wander in "the horizon beyond which [medicine] can not see or say" (Greco, 1998, 71–72). "It [life] return[ed] from its puzzling . . . aliveness to the . . . 'familiar' state of [just another] body within the world of [inanimate material] bodies" (Jonas, 1966, 12). "Death," Jonas concludes, "had [finally] conquered external reality" (13, 15).

It isn't necessary for us to detail what Mary Roach has called "the curious lives of human cadavers" in medical education (Roach, 2003). There was the frantic search for corpses to meet classroom demand following the establishment of the new teaching hospitals in Europe after 1800. There was the rise of an elaborate underground industry of "resurrectionists" (body snatchers) to obtain them, and the generation of an outrageous moral casuistry that permitted the bodies of executed criminals and the poor to be exhumed and dissected for medical purposes. Finally, there were the righteous justifications offered for the practice: "he must mangle the living if he has not first operated on the dead" (says Sir Astley Cooper, surgeon, [Roach, 2003, 46]).[8] What *is* worth noting is that even today, to the most scientifically trained medical student, a "sensed relic," "a faint but telling reminder" of life still dwells in the corpse (Zaner, 1981,

57–58, 65–68). This explains the "gallows humor" of the anatomy lab, a not always successful attempt to defuse the tension that arises when students are confronted by the corpse's hands, face, or genitals.[9] In the end, however, the successful pupil learns the required lesson: when it comes to matters of the body and its ailments, *Körper* is the final tribunal.[10]

Disease

The practice of modern medicine is informed by several disease models. One of them is technically known as monomorphic germ theory. It is the idea that each disease is caused by a specific germ type. While until around 1900 monomorphism was a relatively novel way to view disease, it has since become an essential article of faith for urban, middle-class Euro-Americans. Our goal in the following discussion is to unsettle this conviction.

We begin by reminding ourselves that while monomorphism is thoroughly entrenched in modern consciousness, it is in fact merely one of countless ways to interpret the vague complaints that bring patients to healers. Thus, while it may reveal certain facets of unease, it also precludes alternative ways of seeing and thinking about suffering to those committed to it. Among the virtually countless other ways are chiropracty, shamanism, acupuncture, kahuna, aryu-vedic medicine, and Christian science. All of these disciplines school their practitioners to see the afflictions of human flesh differently than doctors of medicine (M.D.s).

In this century, the most formidable challenge to monomorphism comes from pleomorphism, the paradigm informing naturopathy.[11] We will return to the differences between these two viewpoints momentarily, but first some observations on what they share. Most importantly, both monomorphism and pleomorphism posit that human life is essentially reducible to organic functioning. Both, in other words, are committed to an ontology of the *Körper*. Second, both believe that the presence of disease is signified by organic (cellular) pathologies in the *Körper*. Third, both posit the existence of a causal association between these cellular abnormalities and microscopic particles called germs, to which they attach many of the same labels: bacterium, virus, prion, mold, protozoan, yeast, algae, and so on. What they disagree on is the precise nature and direction of this causal connection. Monomorphs insist that germs cause disease, while pleomorphs argue to the contrary—that disease causes germs. This disagreement has profound implications for how disease is to be treated. Concerning the fact that bodily afflictions *are* problems, however, solvable through the application of scientific principles: M.D.s and naturopaths (N.D.s) are in complete consensus.

Monomorphism

According to monomorphism, there are three necessary and sufficient conditions for disease: a specific microbial agent (i.e., a germ), the vulnerability of an organism to infection by it, and some means to convey that agent to the organism—a vector (from Latin *vehere* = to carry) such as water, food, air, sewage, a rodent or insect, or perhaps a lover's body fluids (Bakalar, 2003). Monomorphs concede that even if an organism is exposed to or even harbors an otherwise deadly germ, say a diphtheria bacilli, *Staphylococcus*, or the retrovirus known as HIV, it may remain disease-free if that germ is unable to break through the organism's defenses. If and when it does, however, the germ will retain its structure throughout the course of the disease.

The title, "monomorphism," is derived from the doctrine of specific etiology, which is attributed to the chemist Robert Koch (1843–1910): for each disease there is one and only one causative germ. According to the rules of bacteriological inquiry first formulated by Koch, in order to prove that a purported germ is indeed causing a disease, the germ must be shown to *always* be present with the disease, present only with *that* disease, and *never* present when there is no disease. Following this logic, rikettsiales, a parasite with a structure similar to a bacterium but without its reproductive capacity, can be considered the cause of typhus; the mosquito-borne protozoan called *Plasmodium*, the cause of malaria; a screw-shaped bacterium known as *Treponema pallidum*, of syphilis; *Vibrio cholerae*, of cholera, and so on. During the nineteenth and twentieth centuries scores of germ-caused diseases were identified (for a sample listing, see Dubos, 1994 [1960], 103). The third generation of monomorphs has since extended germ theory to include atherosclerosis, which they attribute to *Chlamydia pneumoniae* (Sardi, 2006); duodenal ulcers, which are said to be caused by the water-borne bacterium *Helicobacter pylori*; and to a variety of cancers. Enthusiasts now boldly predict that eventually the germs responsible for all known human ailments will be discovered (Hopper, 1999). Obesity, some have suggested, will be found to be caused by virus Ad-36, the same microbe implicated in colds and pinkeye (Salon .com, 2000); female promiscuity, by a parasite named *Toxoplasma gondii* (Bunce, 2006); pediatric obsession, by a type of *Streptococcus* (Hopper, 1999, 50). Although it has yet to be identified, even homosexuality is thought by some to be caused by a germ (Crain, 1999).

Standard hagiographies of germ theory trace it back to the experiments of French chemist Louis Pasteur (1822–1895). Pasteur demonstrated that the souring of milk and the fermentation of grapes into wine were due not to spontaneous generation, but to the effect of yeasts (i.e., germs) on sugar (Duclaux, 1920). Souring and fermentation, in other words, were not the results of the internal chemistries of milk and grapes, but of contact with them of external, minute life forms, which Pasteur originally called "ferments." "The role of the infinitely small in nature," he concluded, "is infinitely large" (Dubos, 1994 [1960], 69). Pasteur went on to argue that fermentation is analogous to the disease process. In fact he wrote of wine fermentation as *les maladie des vin* (the disease of wine).

A close examination of the historical record reveals that Pasteur was not, in fact, the father of germ theory. Three centuries earlier, Hieronymous Fracastoro (in 1546) had argued that poxes, rabies, leprosy, and other contagions were the result of what he named *seminaria*, imperceptible seeds, acquirable either by direct contact or through airborne contamination (Tempkin, 1977, 463). Fracastoro is credited for the naming of syphilis after a character drawn from one of his lyric poems who is destroyed by the gods for impiety. And there were others prior to Fracastoro, for instance, the Roman horticulturist Marcus Terentius Varro (116–27 BCE), who wrote of minute *animalcula* "which by mouth and through the air enter the body and cause severe disease" (Tempkin, 1977, 426–27). In any case, it wasn't until 1884 that one of these hypothesized creatures, now known as a bacterium, was rendered capable of being seen through a microscope. It took five more decades, and the invention of the more powerful electron microscope, before an even tinier particle, the virus, could be observed.

In orthodox epidemiology it is common to read the parable about the "guest-germ" who is "hosted" by a "fertile," infection-prone organism. A more popular allegory is that of battle, wherein the germ is written of as an "alien invader" (cf. Baldry, 1976 [1965]). If the organism's "body armor" is compromised, goes the story (say, by lack of rest, inadequate nutrition, a genetic weakness, abuse of a body part, old age, another preexisting disease, or by inadequate monitoring of the body's "invasion routes," [its pores, nose, eyes, ears, mouth, anus, genitals, or a gaping wound]), then it is susceptible to infection. That is, it is available for being befouled or "stained" by the contaminating agent.

Defeating the enemy involves three tactics. First are defensive measures, of which there are two basic types. One entails girding the body for combat. This involves "training" it ahead of time to identify alien invaders as threats by vaccinating it with their non-lethal cousins. Immunology holds that once successfully tutored, the organism's white blood cells will destroy deadly intruders by engulfing them, a process known as leukocytic phagocytosis. The practice of vaccination was first attempted by Edward Jenner (1749–1823) as a deterrent against smallpox. Using serum derived from running cowpox pustules, vaccination enabled the body to build up antibodies to the far more deadly smallpox bacterium. After witnessing its success in preventing smallpox, the practice was eagerly taken up by Pasteur to deter anthrax and rabies.[12]

A second defensive policy addresses enemy logistics. Here the effort entails interdicting the supply lines, so to say, the vectors that germs utilize to reach the organism's gates. This can include anything from mass flight from a contagious area, to water purification, sanitary sewage disposal, pest control, needle exchanges, condoms, or isolation and quarantining. ("Quarantine" comes from the Latin word for forty. Originally, it referred to the forty days during which a vessel suspected of carrying a disease would be detained in port.)

The tactic of interdiction rarely achieves the notoriety of a Koch, a Pasteur, or a Rudolf Virchow, three heroes in the pantheon of monomorphism, all of whom are mythologized as devotedly laboring away alone in their laboratories (cf. De Kruif, 1959 [1926]; Metchinkoff, 1971 [1939]). Nonetheless, apart from a handful of cases like smallpox and polio, interdiction has played a far greater role in reducing death from infection than either immunization or the offensive tactics discussed below. Indeed, research shows that in America since 1900 only about 5 percent of the drop in mortality rates from measles, tuberculosis, scarlet fever, influenza, pneumonia, diphtheria, whooping cough, and typhoid fever can be attributed to standard medical intervention (McKinlay and McKinlay, 1994). Instead, it is due primarily to the introduction of public sewage and garbage disposal systems, sanitary water supplies, better nutritional practices, health education, pollution abatement, and occupational safety laws.

An effective campaign against germs also requires the deployment of offensive weaponry, most importantly "guided missiles" or "magic bullets," the latter a figure of speech coined by the father of chemotherapy, early twentieth-century German chemist Paul Ehrlich. Among them are sulphonamides (made from Ehrlich's aniline dyes), penicillins (from molds), streptomycins (from soil), cephalosporins (from sea algae), and others like quinine, which is derived from seeds of the cinchona tree.

Besides magic bullets are two other offensive tactics. One is tactical retreat, so to speak, the ceding of already diseased or dead tissue to the enemy through surgical extirpation. Another is a variation on the scorched earth policy: radiating or cauterizing the infection, or applying hydrogen peroxide or carbolic acid (phenol) to it.[13] It is through the poisoning, cutting, and burning of recalcitrant flesh in the operating room or hospital radiation department that physicians and patients are reminded that modern medicine is like military science. And like war, the struggle against disease calls for courage, persistence, and, occasionally, coldhearted discipline.

Orthodox medicine's strategy for fighting disease is constantly being refined and revised, yet the theory underlying it, technically known as allopathy, has a centuries-old Greek pedigree. Expressed in the Latin phrase *contraria contrariis sanantur*, it is that contraries are best cured by contraries, the pains of disease by equal and opposite doses of remedial pain. This theory in turn is based on the idea that health is a kind of equilibrium. Originally, this referred to a balance between the so-called humors once considered elemental to life. For the Greek physician, Hippocrates, these were blood, phlegm, and yellow and black biles.

Allopathy was imported into Western Europe by itinerant Celtic monks who had labored in Syrian monastic hospitals from around 300 to 600 CE. It came to constitute not only the basis of modern medical therapy, but also the underpinnings for the Roman Catholic sacrament of penance (J. Aho, 2005, 13–18). Even today, priests are routinely spoken of as administering *medicamenta* or *fomenta* (poultices) to "remedy" the "spiritual infirmities" of their "patients" (Denzinger, 1957, 173, secs. 437, 274–79, 879–906). Medieval confessional handbooks actually went so far as to attribute specific physical afflictions to their supposed sinful causes. Heart disease was said to be due to pride, for example, frenzy to anger, leprosy to envy, and epilepsy to lechery (McNeill, 1932).

The penances prescribed by "spiritual physicians" for *cura animarum* (cure of the soul) were often brutal. They could range anywhere from sleep deprivation, cold-water baths, fasting, and the application of stinging nettles to blood-soaking flagellation, solitary confinement, and exile. Likewise, the original allopathic medical treatments: they typically involved bloodletting, forced vomiting, enemas, and sweating. These were painful and dangerous, often purposively so. This was especially true for venereal diseases, which, as the name suggests, were considered products of venery, evil. "It [syphilis] is never resolved," asserts an early commentator on the subject, "except under the influence of a medication which imposes on the body the chastisement of its impurity and on the soul the punishment of its error" (Tempkin, 1977, 475). The medication of which he speaks is mercury, which induces sweating. To be effective, the mercury cure (or punishment, as the case may be) was supposed to produce a gallon of liquid daily for a month. We can understand why, until after 1900 when doctors adopted anesthesia and antiseptics, those who could afford to do so avoided making appointments with the local allopath. (As a period satire taught, notwithstanding the heroic measures undertaken by M.D.s, sometimes "nature gets the better of the Doctor, and the patient recovers" [Ehrenreich and English, 2005, 49]). Even today physician-induced (iatrogenic) fatality is a leading cause of death in America. The majority of these are due to adverse reactions from properly administered drugs (Lazarou et al., 1998).

While it will take us too far afield to address the question in any depth, it is worth asking how, if this is true, did allopathic physicians (i.e., M.D.s) come to assume a virtual monopoly over the administration of bodily care in America during the last century. The short answer is that it was through the organizational discipline of the chief lobby of medical doctors, the American Medical Association (AMA), which was founded in 1870 (Starr, 1982). By shrewdly staging itself as a defender of free-market capitalism, community-oriented altruism, and science-based technical proficiency, the AMA was able to co-opt psychiatrists, radiologists, pharmacists, and surgeons into becoming its allies. It then set about marginalizing other potential competitors as self-serving quacks, making it illegal for them to advertise themselves as health care providers. These included midwives, homeopathic physicians, chiropractors, herbalists, bonesetters, horse doctors, patent medicine peddlers, and barbers (Ehrenreich and English, 2005, 76–108).[14]

Yet all is not well with medical orthodoxy. In the words of one of its celebrants, "man's discovery of antimicrobial agents must surely rank as one of his [sic] greatest triumphs" (Baldry, 1976 [1965], 156). He then continues on to admit that "a spirit of disillusionment" has nonetheless settled over the profession.

This is because of growing "enemy resistance" to its campaign strategy. Germs once thought to be permanently defeated are rebounding with renewed ferocity, and "no one should underestimate [their] cunning" (156). As strains of penicillin-sensitive *Staphylococci* were eliminated, the survivors rearmed themselves with a capacity to excrete penicillianase, a toxin that counteracts the drug's medicinal effect. The result: "flesh-eating" staph (MRSA = methicillin-resistant *Staphylococcus aureus*).

At first penicillin-resistant infections were of little concern because it was thought they could be treated with alternative antibiotics. Now, however, germs have evolved that display immunity to all known magic bullets: antibiotic-resistant tuberculosis viruses, rapidly mutating HIV, ebola, gonorrhea, and so on. MRSA alone is estimated to have infected and killed more Americans in 2005 than AIDS (Klevens et al., 2007). Like phoenixes rising from fires lit to kill them, we are witnessing the "the revenge of the microbes" (Salyers and Whitt, 2005). "Super bugs," virulent versions of germs once thought to be eliminated, are emerging from the charred husks of their dead cousins. This has necessitated wholesale rethinking of the battle strategy of frontally attacking germs with a medical version of total war. Instead, a more selective, precisely targeted, some even call it "diplomatic," response to alien invaders is in the process of being implemented (Baldry, 1976 [1965], 170–71). Drug resistance has also opened the door to another, heterodox, way of conceiving disease. That other way is pleomorphism.

Pleomorphism

According to pleomorhpism, the precursors to all living matter are *microzymae* (Gr. = little bodies), simple proteins within cells that ferment (digest) naturally produced body sugars (Bird, n.db.; Bird, 1991; Baker, 1994).[15] When the cells are healthy, these tiny beings quietly go about their business. However, if the ph level (acidity) of the cells rises beyond a particular point, if the cells exhibit the incorrect electromagnetic charge, or have low oxygen concentrations, then the microzymae can become "morbid." They can morph successively into viruses, bacteria, and ultimately, into molds. That is to say, they can become germs. The word for this process is "pleomorphism," a term coined by Pasteur's one-time assistant and later archrival, Antoine Béchamp (1816–1908). Béchamp claims that as germs start to digest unhealthy cellular material, they exude their own toxic wastes. This is known as mycotoxicosis. It is mycotoxicosis that produces the symptoms associated with disease, not the germ itself. Indeed there are no specific diseases, according to pleomorphs. There are only general symptoms—fever, pain, tumors, fatigue, foul odors, swelling, diarrhea, and so on—that reflect the pathology of the body's cells.

While during his lifetime Béchamp was a celebrated pharmacist and biochemist, after his death he was forgotten. Pleomorphs suspect that this is due to monomorphic treachery, a view since partially confirmed by renowned historian of science Gerald Geison (1995, 267).[16] Geison contrasts Béchamp's postmortem fate with that of Pasteur, which he claims was prepared ahead of time by Pasteur himself and his family. In any case, following his death Pasteur was given full military honors in a ceremony attended by the president of the Third Republic on what was announced as a national day of mourning. *Un bienfaiteur de l'humanite*, read the posters along the parade route, *Pasteur est eternal*. "A benefactor of humanity"; "Pasteur is immortal" (Geison, 1995, 259; plates 21 and 22). He was subsequently memorialized with the names of boulevards, schools, hospitals, and laboratories throughout the world, as well as in songs, homilies, and in an Oscar-winning movie. His advocates in fact once proposed that an entire region of French colonial Africa be retitled "Pastoria" after their hero (Geison, 1995, 262). Meanwhile, Béchamp's name was expunged from official histories of modern medicine (Nonclercq, 1978).

In the hands of Béchamp's protégés, the battle metaphor for dealing with disease is senseless, for germs are not considered tiny foreign agents trying to breach the walls of the body fortress. On the contrary, they are "nature's scavengers," endogenous "janitors" that sweep away the rubbish of dead and dying cellular matter. Thus, disease is not so much a thing to be "fought" as it is a condition to be prevented. And not by "artificial" allopathic means, but naturally, by assisting the patient to maintain the integrity of their "inner terrain" (cf. Appleton, 1999). This includes cleansing the system of toxic wastes, maintaining a proper cellular acid-base balance, and keeping the cells adequately fed. In short, deal with disease by "getting rid of the garbage that attracts flies."

Garbage removal requires a variety of actions. First is the regular consumption of "green juices" and high fiber colon cleansers, together with at least eight glasses of distilled water daily. It is recommended that this be accompanied by periodic "internal baths" (enemas) using either lemon juice or coffee. Severe cases of cellular toxication may call for oral or intravenous chelation treatments. Chelators are compounds like sea kelp, chromium, and EDTA that presumably bind with toxic heavy metals in the body like lead or depleted uranium, or with arterial calcium plaques. These are subsequently excreted in urine. A second preventative measure consists of daily sessions of aerobic exercise coupled with meditative deep breathing using the diaphragm instead of the upper chest. These have obvious oxygenizing benefits, but they are also stress relievers. High chronic levels of stress-related cortisol and adrenaline are considered toxic to cells. Third is a vegan diet of "basic" (non-acidic), "live" (uncooked), "organic" (non-pesticide or insecticide) vegetables, fruits, whole grains, and nuts. The consumption of red meat, considered an acidic substance, is discouraged. Earth-resonant herbal teas and selected barks, stems, seeds, and flower supplements, on the other hand, are highly recommended (Balch, 2006). As, furthermore, is the consumption of "probiotics." These are germs such as *bifidobacteria* and *lactobacilli*, which are widely known to aid digestion, and are found in non-pasteurized yogurt and milk.

All this probably screams "new age!" to readers. However, the naturopathic regimen, like allopathy, has its own age-old precursors. A healthy diet for Hippocrates did not refer to caloric intake, a measure of energy that betrays the modern custom of reducing life to organic functioning, but to one's total way of inhabiting the world. Only through a proper diet of eating and vomiting, vigorous athletics, moderate pleasure-seeking, plus the love of wisdom (i.e., philosophy), it was taught, could one hope to attain the balance of humors believed essential for health and well-being.

Licensed pharmaceutical firms devise, test, and sell the arsenal of treatments alluded to above, utilized by monomorphs in their battle against infection. Pleomorphs have an equally imposing (if not nearly as capitalized) industrial arm, nutraceutical manufacturing. Nutraceuticals are edible substances that are neither foods nor drugs, but occupy a limbo outside oversight of the Food and Drug Administration (FDA) (Specter, 2004). This is because instead of claiming that they cure specific diseases, which would legally require double-blind experimental confirmation, nutraceuticals are sold as offering "hope" to the overweight and "prevention" against the ravages of time. And insofar as nutraceuticals are not strictly foods, their purity need not be attested to by independent government laboratories. In fact, there exists some concern that at least a few of the concoctions are dangerous (Palmer, 2006).

America has a long, colorful history of patent medicines like Lydia Pinkham's Vegetable Compound (made up mostly of alcohol and vegetable extracts), Coca-Cola (originally made in part from the coca leaf), and reputed health foods like Sylvester Graham's crackers and W. W. Kellogg's cereals. It is a history rooted in the American public hygiene movement of the nineteenth century, which was originally headquartered in the Yankee states of New England and the Old Northwest. Today, one of the centers of the nutraceutical industry is along the Wasatch Front in Utah and Idaho, or, as it is locally called, "Cellulose Valley." Many natural supplement companies such as Basic Research, Pure Fruit Technologies Inc., MonaVie, and Utah Scientific are owned by Church of Jesus Christ of Latter-day Saint (Mormon) elders. The Mormon "Word of Wisdom" (authored ca. 1833) praises "herbs and roots," grains, and "every fruit," for their God-bestowed health benefits, while it berates "fermented grape," "strong drinks," and tobacco (Doctrine and Covenants, sec. 89). The first Mormon nutraceutical firms were established in the 1940s. Typically they employ multilevel marketing techniques whereby independent contractors earn commissions for items they sell, plus payouts on earnings from others they have enlisted as distributors. Trained in door-to-door evangelism, Mormons make talented salespeople.

Pleomorphs claim that the reputed wonder drugs of conventional medicine do not actually cure disease. Quite the contrary, they merely change the conditions of the cells, often to the organism's detriment. A case in point is childhood inoculations, the sera of which are derived from infected cows, chickens, pigs, or horses, and which are (or at least used to be) preserved in mercury or formaldehyde (Peters, 1993; McBeam, 1974 [1957]).

According to pleomorphs, the autoimmune conditions of lupus and rheumatoid arthritis are actually delayed anaphylactic responses of microzymae to foreign proteins that were earlier injected into the patient's body via inoculation. A similar explanation is given for dementias like Parkinson's and Alzheimer's, for angina and edema, as well as for liver cirrhosis and jaundice. The alleged epidemic of sudden infant death syndrome (SIDS) cases, childhood autism, dyslexia, and growing numbers of childhood ODD and ADHD diagnoses are accounted for the same way, as is the explosion of cancers during the last century. Cancer, say pleomorphs, is a systematic (general cellular) condition that localizes in a particular organ, not a local disease that metastasizes (Bird, 1991, 21). Its ultimate cause is neither infection nor genetic mutation, but mycotoxicosis. Likewise, AIDS. Reasonable pleomorphs concede that "the best and most certain way to prevent AIDS is to avoid exchanging bodily fluids with people who are HIV+." However, they insist that the most effective countermeasure against AIDS is not the antiviral medicine AZT, but naturopathic "tonification" of the body's immune system (Ullman, 1995).

This being the case, pleomorphs have come to question the wisdom of compulsory childhood vaccination programs. Some, admittedly extreme, pleomorphs consider such programs to be phases in a secret plan by AMA "poison squirters" to weaken the body politic, making it susceptible to the machinations of a secret cabal like the New World Order or, more menacingly, to ZOG, Zionist Occupation Government.[17] Moderate pleomorphs agree that there is a conspiracy, but they believe that its purpose is purely mercenary, to line the pockets of pharmaceutical companies at the expense of the nation's health (Illich, 1976). Either way, pleomorphism is far more than just a theory of disease. It is a component of a larger ideological movement that promotes self-reliance in the face of the increasingly centralized bureaucratic regimentation of health care by mainstream biomedicine. This explains its attraction to, among other marginalized constituencies, religious fundamentalists, as well as to romantic leftists, both of whom place a premium on individual responsibility. It remains an open question whether consumers of naturopathy are in fact less vulnerable to financial abuse (or physical danger) when they place their well-being in the hands of pleomorphs rather than in those of medical doctors.

Negotiating the Dispute

According to Nietzsche, there is no truth. All that exist are truth *claims*, the unending play of different narratives and perspectives. "What, then, is truth?" he once asked. "A mobile army of metaphors, metonyms, and anthropomorphisms . . . embellished poetically and rhetorically, and which after long use seem firm, canonical, and obligatory to a people" (Nietzsche, 1968 [1954], 46–47). Edmund Husserl, the father of phenomenology, was deeply suspicious of Nietzsche's indictment of foundational truth claims and his seeming endorsement of irrationality.[18] Nevertheless, at least in its existentialist and postmodern varieties, phenomenology is indebted to Nietzsche's unsparing critique of the possibility of discovering timeless objective truths. By the same token, however, it may also be considered the source of phenomenology's enduring weakness.

When little is at stake the idea of the play of perspectives is a harmless bagatelle: intriguing, perhaps, a little scandalous, and maybe even fun. But when it comes to matters life and death, as in the case of my own cancer or heart disease, my own child's autism, or my own mother's lupus, it can be unsatisfying; some would say, morally intolerable. It may be that the perspectives of monomorphism and pleomorphism are equally "valid" in the

Nietzschean sense. But in matters of disease, we want to know the truth so as to be able to act, and act effectively.[19] In closing, then, here are four comments intended as trail-markers in negotiating the terrain of medical truth claims. Let us begin by reviewing what has already been established above.

Both pleomorphs and monomorphs can trace their ancestries back many centuries, and today both labor in shiny laboratories outfitted with glasswear, rubber tubing, and stainless steel instruments. While monomorphs have their beeping, flashing electronic monitors, pleomorphs have their own QXCI (xrroid consciousness interface) machines and monochromatic lasers. Both, furthermore, have access to an impressive array of media outlets to disseminate their views: pleomorphs, primarily marginal alternative book publishers and the Internet; monomorphs, mainline refereed academic and professional journals. In these, each mounts stinging rebukes of the other, accusing each other of fostering diseases on a hapless public either out of ignorance, for the sake of money, or worse. Pleomorphs are ridiculed as "charlatans" and "quacks"; monomorphs, as "plagiarists" and "imposters." At the same time, each honors its own stable of persecuted prophets: monomorphs, Ignaz Semmelweis and Jonathan Snow; pleomorphs, Royal Rife and Gaston Naessens. Our first point is this: no matter how aesthetically attractive and emotionally moving these ploys and devices are, none bear on the soundness of pleomorphism or monomorphism. To assess this requires an independent criterion of justifiability.

Our second point concerns what exactly this standard should be. One possibility is clear: confirmation. Which of the two theories is more highly verified? Unfortunately, while such a rule seems intuitively obvious, it leads to an impasse, for both pleomorphs and monomorphs boast of enjoying lavish factual support.[20] This is hardly unique to medical science. Karl Popper long ago showed that one can find "evidence" for virtually any hypothesis, including that the earth is the center of the universe or that the earth is flat. In the latter case, all one need do is ascend a local hill on a clear day and view the plane of the horizon. Voila! (Popper, 1968). This being so, Popper proposes a minimalist criterion of scientific acceptance: falsifiability. Is the theory in principle capable of being refuted? Can we imagine a test that could conceivably disprove it? If so, then it deserves the title "science." If no, then it is not truly scientific, but merely a self-confirming, circular argument. Armed with this criterion, Popper goes on to show that psychoanalysis, Marxism, fascism, utilitarian economics, and indeed most social theories are in fact pseudo-sciences. They may be posed in Greek terminology, mathematical symbols, and acronyms, but they explain little, if anything.[21] This brings us to a third point.

Monomorphs deride pleomorphs for their evident inability to account for contagions: cholera epidemics, the scourge of polio, tuberculosis outbreaks, and so on. Pleomorphs reply by arguing that monomorphism is powerless to explain why it is that even when the presumed germs for these diseases are known to be flourishing in a population, most people do not get sick from them. Pleomorphs and monomorphs rarely acknowledge the validity of the other's criticism. On the contrary, instead of granting the possibility that their fundamental assumptions about disease causality might be questionable, or at least limited in applicability, each pleads for more time, more money, more patience to address the anomaly. More troubling still is that monomorphs and pleomorphs employ technologies of observation that seem at first glance to foreclose the possibility of their assumptions *ever* being refuted.

Pleomorphs claim that the dyes used to fix blood samples for lab testing, plus the electron microscopes that blast the smears with radiation, kill microzymae. This, they say, makes it impossible to witness the pleomorphic process, the intracellular changes that lead to the formation of minute "janitor germs." What monomorphs witness instead through their lenses is the "dead carnage of the battlefield": an intact cell wall, a nucleus, and degraded germ remnants. This has the effect of "confirming" the monomorphic axiom that behind each disease resides one specific microbe. To overcome this alleged methodological problem, pleomorphs utilize (or at least endorse) a less intrusive observational instrument, the Rife universal optical microscope. By using natural refracted light instead of electronic beams, the Rife microscope presumably allows live blood samples to be viewed.[22] Cellular dynamism becomes visible. In place of dead germs, the pleomorphic process of microzymae evolving successively into viruses, bacteria, and fungi can be witnessed. Assuming they have ever heard of the Rife microscope, which is doubtful, much less seen one, monomorphs would dismiss it as impossible according to the laws of optics, and another example of fakery.

The bottom line is that the relative veracity of monomorphism and pleomorphism to each other is, at least at this point, incapable of being adjudicated by means of a standard both are willing to accept. What this means is that each school of thought is what Thomas Kuhn would call a self-reflexive paradigm: a system of causal laws about disease, a body of classic experiments to "prove" those laws, plus—and this is most important—an accepted set of tools and protocols to observe the experiments (Kuhn, 1970). That monomorphism prevails today in Euro-America is due not just to its laboratory findings and clinical successes (many of which pleomorphs dispute in any case [c.f. McBeam, 1974 (1957)]), but to other, non-scientific considerations, some of which we have already mentioned above.[23]

So we come full circle back to Nietzsche. In regard to the nature, causes, and cures of disease, truth evidently *is* elusive. Both medical orthodoxy and heterodoxy appear to be erected on foundations less solid than popular sentiment would hope. This is not to say that they are hermetically closed off from outside influence. Each can and has in the past profited from the presence of the other.

Ironically, an important case in point is afforded by the reputed father of monomorphism himself, Louis Pasteur. After observing that most silkworms never came down with the diseases caused by the germs that he had discovered, Pasteur confessed that were he to undertake new studies, "I would direct my efforts to the environmental conditions that increase their [the worms'] vigor and resistance. . . . *I am convinced that it would be possible to discover techniques for improving the physiological state of worms and thereby increase their resistance to disease*" (Dubos, 1994 [1960], 133, our italics). As for human pathologies, historian René Dubos claims that the possibility became "almost . . . an obsession" with Pasteur that by manipulating their "inner ter-rain"—a phrase that he might well have adopted from his erst-while enemy, Béchamp—people could be made less susceptible to infection. Included in this so-called terrain, Pasteur believed, are the acid-base balance of the patient's cells and their mental state: their degree of hopefulness and courage (136). One pleo-morphic legend maintains that Pasteur's last words were, "Claude Bernard was right. . . . the microbe is nothing, the ter-rain is everything" (Appleton, 1999, 47).

There are, furthermore, perfectly good reasons why mutual borrowing like this is to be expected. After all, for all their dif-ferences, monomorphs and pleomorphs share an overriding conviction. It is that body troubles, including the ultimate afflic-tion, death, are diseases—cellular abnormalities capable of being "managed" by professional experts. Or, to express it in the re-verse, both monomorphs and pleomorphs are implicated in a project that, by overlooking the experience of illness, threatens to diminish the sufferer (Redding, 1995, 93). This leads to our fourth and final comment.

If phenomenology teaches us but one lesson, it is that the *Körper* provides at best only a shadowy facsimile of life. It does not enable us to understand the concrete experience of living. In other words, a *Körper* is not a *Leib*. It is not alive, not a living per-son. On the contrary, *Leib* is a "hoax" on the *Körper* (a *ludibrium materium*) (Jonas, 1966, 12; Zaner, 1984).

Richard Zaner describes how, after the "the obvious opulence of animate life" was stripped from human flesh during the mod-ern era, beginning with William Harvey's dissections and ending with La Mettrie's proclamation that human flesh is little more than a complex mechanism, something unforeseen began to show up: pathological presentments inexplicable in organic terms. Today, they are familiar to every physician: patients who exhibit debilitating symptoms, but who have no signs of disease, no clinically detectable organic pathology. But there is another, "much more serious" hoax on matter that we want to address here (Toombs, 1992, 19–24; cf. Zaner, 2004). It is the lived agonies of illness: the discredit, anger, pain, confusion, terror, and dimin-ishment undergone by those who *do* have a laboratory-verified disease. For just as human completeness (health) is not the same as physiological normality, and being healed (made whole) is far from identical to being cured, so lived illness is never just a disease.

For half a century E. E. Rosenbaum practiced medicine, convinced that bodily ailments could only be grasped biologically, through the examination of physical lesions. Not until he became ill himself and got "a taste of his own medicine" while lying in a hospital bed did he come to realize how terribly wrong he had been all those years (Rosenbaum, 1988). A "deep chasm," he found, exists between the world of the patient and that of the doctor. He found a "decisive gap" that distorts their communications, frustrates diagnoses, and interferes with effective treatment. Kay Toombs, a philosopher who underwent a similar experience as a victim of multiple sclerosis, agrees. Where the doctors "gazed" at her progressive enfeeblement through the naturalistic lens of science, seeing it variously as either "interesting" or "boring," she was condemned to suffer its humiliations alone. And where many of the doctors' therapies were medically indicated, they sometimes entailed side effects that enhanced her suffering. Her conclusion: "[T]o bypass the patient's voice is to bypass the illness itself." And to bypass the illness is to overlook the patient (Toombs, 1992, 28). This being so, let us follow Toombs's recommendation and give ear to the patient.

Notes

1. In this book, we give the phrase "eidetic essence" a non-Husserlian twist. For us, it refers only to the experiential qualities of diseases, sickness, and illnesses that are themselves culturally and historically conditioned.

2. Eric Cassell, an authority on this subject, maintains that "two generations of attempts to [train doctors to attend to feelings] have had remarkably little effect" (Cassell, 1991, 138).

3. We are not saying that practicing physicians summarily overlook the feelings of their patients. Nor is it that doctors *should* disavow the logic of scientific inquiry and attend more closely to the promptings of their guts when conducting diagnoses (for a cautionary tale, see Groopman, 2007). Rather, it is to argue that the ends of science and the purposes of day-to-day doctoring are not always compatible. The object of medical science is to generate universal laws

of biochemical functioning; the goal of medical practice is to allay personal suffering. Thus, while the science of biomedicine necessarily abjures value judgments, it is precisely informed judiciousness based on years of clinical experience that characterizes a good doctor (Cassell, 1991, 104–8). Eric Cassell decries the widespread conflation of medical science with doctoring, and the belief shared by more and more young physicians that it is scientific technology that cures, not they themselves.

4. That is, the displacement of an object to a distance of one centimeter by one dyne of propulsive force.

5. It is ironic that in his critique of materialistic culture, Jonas himself defines life in terms of biological metabolism. For a thoroughgoing critique of this move by one of his protégés, see Zaner (1981, 6–22).

6. Translated into English in 1749.

7. For more on the romantic revolt against scientism, see the appendix.

8. In point of fact, neither the founder of Chinese medicine, Huang Ti (fl. ca. 2600 BCE), his Western counterpart, Hippocrates, nor the renowned Greco-Roman anatomist, Galen, endorsed dissection (Roach, 2003, 52–54).

9. Most students overcome their hesitations through depersonalization, that is, by forcing themselves to think of the organs as dead tissue, not as once-living flesh. Others, failing this, have been observed to place white linen napkins over cadaver heads, of assuming an attitude of reverence toward "their" bodies, of personalizing them with names, or of even holding perfunctory memorial services in their behalf (Roach, 2003, 37–39).

10. Besides its use in gross anatomy labs, one of the most telling reflections of the significance of the corpse in our era is its use as an object of interrogation in medical forensics, as indicated in the wildly popular TV series *CSI: Crime Scene Investigation*. The potassium level of a dead body, its temperature, the age of its fly larvae, the degree of its epidermal slough-age, the extent of its organ bloating, and its "odor signatures" can, like printed texts, be read like a victim's diary and then deployed in courtrooms, becoming the last word, not only on the time of death, but its cause (Bass and Jefferson, 2004).

11. In oncology, a specialty in medical orthodoxy, "pleomorphism" refers to highly variable cell nuclei in cancerous cells. As will be clear later, naturopaths use the term very differently.

12. Lady Mary Wortley, wife of the English ambassador to Turkey, experimented with vaccinations as early as 1717. Inoculation against smallpox had already long been practiced in Turkey.

13. Introduced by Scottish surgeon Joseph Lister (1827–1912), phenol was the first modern antiseptic. Lister is credited for making the connection between the suppuration of wounds and fermentation.

14. The red and white stripes of the barber's pole originally stood for the bandages stained from bloodletting; the brass basins on its top and bottom, respectively, to the leech container and blood receptacle. The pole itself referred to what patients gripped to encourage blood flow.

15. There are scores of websites on pleomorphism. Besides those cited in the text are these: www.educate-yourself.org/cn/pleomorphismdiscovery suppression16; www.rawplaeodiet.org/pleomorphism-1; and hbci.com/~wenonah/new/naessens. Some of these sites also access subscribers to subjects like ancient astronauts, aromatherapy, chakra healing, the hydrazine sulfate cure, a mysterious substance known as 714-X, Sumerian clothing, and conspiratology.

16. The original indictment has been "reassembled," says Geison, numerous times, most notably by R. B. Pearson in his 1942 alternative health cult classic, *Pasteur: Plagarist, Imposter* (Pearson, 1942). A book review of the original version, written by an apologist for monomorphism, ends with the following claim: "The emotional basis, the intellectual feebleness, and the anti-social character of the whole anti-medical movement is superbly illustrated in the motivation and in the pseudo-scientific and oft times painfully unintelligent contents of this subsidized book of propaganda" (C. A. K., 1934).

17. In 1919 William F. Koch introduced a pill of still undetermined composition called Glyoxilide. Koch claimed that by oxygenating the cells, it could cure cancer. Allegedly because it worked so well, rendering hospitals, pharmaceuticals, and health insurance superfluous, "Jewish medical demagogues" sought to criminalize its use (Hunt, 1976). For the persecution of pleomorph Gaston Naessens, see Bird (1991).

18. Husserl believed that by means of phenomenological inquiry, investigators could access the "apodictic [indubitable] features" of the transcendental ego; the presumed universal, transhistorical structures that make meaningful experience possible.

19. For a riveting depiction of the stakes involved in the dispute over the causes of AIDS, see Specter (2007).

20. For one example, see the admittedly self-serving account by Harry Hoxsey of his experiments on a cancer cure (Hoxsey, 1956). See also Anonymous (1956).

21. "'Science, no less than any other form of culture, depends on rhetoric.' And superficially anti-rhetorical language of most modern science is itself but another rhetorical . . . strategy" (Geison, 1995, 269).

22. According to advocates, the Rife microscope has a magnifying power of sixty thousand times greater than what can be seen through clear glass. This allegedly enabled its inventor to observe the BX virus, which he claimed was associated with (but did not cause) all cancers. For excellent photos of the microscope as well as several of its images, see Xenophilia (2003). For other accounts of this technology, see Beardon (n.d.) and Bird (n.da.). Originally a researcher at the University of Southern California, Rife was hounded out of academia, landed in an insane asylum, and eventually disappeared.

23. For characterization of orthodox germ theory as a religion, see Smith (2005). An earlier example on this same line is Dresden (1931).

6

The Agonies of Illness

How are we when we are ill? This is our concern in this chapter. Before addressing the subject, several caveats are in order.

There is, of course, a multiplicity of illnesses. Some, like the measles or a cold, are acute and self-limiting; others are chronic. Of the latter, some are minimally disruptive and are treated relatively inexpensively; others can eat into a family's economic sustenance as they cripple their victim. Long-lasting, debilitating, and deadly afflictions often are most disclosive of the precariousness and contingency of human existence (although acute diseases like kidney stones or appendicitis may have comparable impacts). Hence, they lend themselves best to our kind phenomenological inquiry. It is primarily those, therefore, that we focus on here.

It is important to stress at the outset that our account should in no way be taken as a causal explanation of illness. While in the last chapter we saw that issues of causality are important, the goal of phenomenology is to return "to the things themselves." Or, to express the same point in terms introduced earlier, our concern in the following discussion is not so much with the pathologies of the *Körper* as with the experiences of *Leib*.

Because scientific methodology is thought by phenomenologists to distort the ways that things show themselves in lived experience, phenomenology tries to suspend or "bracket out" assumptions of detached objectivity and presumptions of causality. Instead, it attends to the ways by which things—in this case, illness—are typically *experienced*. We enter these experiences by drawing on first-person narratives of the ill. No claim is made that every person lives illness in exactly the same way. For purposes of convenience we simply ignore the countless differences by which the general themes enumerated below can be and are colored by age, gender, and religious, historical, and geographic factors. Nor do we deny that analysts coming at illness from a standpoint other than ours might see illness differently than we.

The Body's Disappearance and Appearance

A good place to start is with Heidegger's classic work, *Being and Time* (1962), a book that actually says very little about the body, health, or illness, but offers a groundbreaking analysis of how we comport with what he calls "tools" or "equipment" (*Zeugen*). By this he means houses, offices, cars, computers, cell phones, and the like: things that we are already involved with and handle every day. What makes Heidegger's account helpful for our purposes is that it undermines the scientific interpretation of things as isolated objects held under the theoretical gaze of a knowing subject. According to Heidegger, in the course of our workday acts and practices, there is no detached standpoint from which objects are observed. Rather, we are already engaged with them as we go about our tasks. They are "handy" (*zuhanden*). The car gets me to work, the key opens the office door, and the computer sends e-mail. In other words, we understand these things not by studying them or staring at them as a scientist might do, but by *using* them.

Heidegger's second point is that we are never involved with just a single piece of equipment. We never understand tools in isolation. On the contrary, they come to us as components of an interconnected totality of other tools. "There 'is' no such thing as *an* equipment," he says. Rather, "equipment is always in terms of its belonging to other equipment" (Heidegger, 1962, 68). A car has no meaning outside the context of a street with speed signs and bumps, mall parking lots, photo IDs, gas stations, convenience stores, and service people. And vice versa—none of the latter makes much sense without cars. In fact on closer view, none of these are understandable outside the context of the entire modern urban world.

In Heidegger's view, we "grow into" a shared familiarity of equipmental contexts, and once we are absorbed we are no longer thematically aware of the tools themselves. I don't conduct a cost/benefit analysis before choosing a lane in which to drive on my way to work in the morning. I simply find myself on the right side of the road (assuming, of course, that I am an American). Likewise, we open doors and type on computers without being explicitly aware of the doorknobs or keyboards. In the prereflective flow and rhythm of everydayness, we are woven into the world in such a way that the tools have a tendency to disappear or "withdraw" (*zurückziehen*) (Heidegger, 1962, 99).

Our bodies can also be understood as a complex of instruments, each of which serves a particular purpose. In fact, Heidegger traces the word "organ" to the Greek *organon*, which means, precisely, instrument or tool. "The [bodily] organ is a *Werkzeug*," he says, "a working instrument" (Heidegger, 1995, 213). Like the other equipment that surrounds us, our organs are always already busy at work: digesting, breathing, seeing, hearing, walking, and so forth. And just as I do not normally notice the keyboard, the desk, or the chair as I type my notes on the computer, when my organs are laboring smoothly, my body "hides" itself. I am not aware of my heart, lungs, legs, and arms as I walk down the hallway with my briefcase (Cerbone, 2000, 218–19). Heidegger's student, Hans-Georg Gadamer, describes this state of hidden bodying-forth (*Leiben*) as "health."

> So what possibilities stand before us when we are considering the question of health? Without doubt it is part of our nature as living beings that our conscious self-awareness remains largely in the background so that our enjoyment of good health is constantly concealed from us. Yet despite its hidden character

health none the less manifests itself in a general feeling of well-being. It shows itself above all where such a feeling of well-being means we are open to new things, ready to embark on new enterprises and, forgetful of ourselves, scarcely notic[ing] the demands and strains which are put on us. This is what health is. (Gadamer, 1996, 112)

When we are healthily and rhythmically engaged in worldly tasks our bodies "disappear." Heidegger calls this condition "everydayness" (*Alltäglichkeit*). In the state of everydayness, things go well; they fit together as they should. Fredrik Svenaeus, following Heidegger's lead, prefers the word "homelikeness," which he describes as "a rhythmic, balancing mood that supports our understanding in a homelike way without calling for our attention" (Svenaeus, 2000, 94).

Heidegger goes on to say that this mode of awareness shifts when tools malfunction. When the front door fails to open as I insert the house key, my familiar prereflective bond with the world breaks and the key emerges from its invisibility *as* a key. I am suddenly a detached knower examining the objective properties of the knob, the keychain, and my hands. Once I find the correct key, insert it, and the door opens, this momentary subject/object split dissolves; just as quickly I am reabsorbed into the flow of everydayness. I am "home" again.

Something similar occurs with our body parts. We become explicitly aware of our stomach, for example, wrist, or knee at the very instant that their taken-for-granted reliability breaks down. In the exact moment that their function is "lost," says Heidegger, they are "found" (Heidegger, 1962, 126–27, 164; Sartre, 1956, 436–41; Toombs, 1992, 33–38, 51–52).

Having said this, Heidegger acknowledges an important difference between a tool and a bodily organ. A hammer or a book is something that has an existence outside and independent from me, and is thus available for use by others. An organ, in contrast, belongs to me and me alone as a "unique and singular living being" (Heidegger, 1995, 219; McNeill, 2006, 6). What he would say in light of the emerging enterprise of organ donation must remain unanswered. But ignoring this question, what Heidegger is getting at is that while a neighbor might borrow my lawnmower, s/he can never share my illness. No one can experience the way *I* am pulled out of the easeful pace of daily life and thrust into dis-ease, where the world no longer makes sense in the way it used to, and my body becomes an alien burden.

Pain

There is probably nothing that makes me more aware of my body than pain. It is the major reason why people make appointments to see the doctor. But *how* is pain? There was the British farmer caught in a hay baler. Fearful that his entire body would be dragged in and crushed, he amputated his hand with a three-inch pocketknife. Then, there was the American outdoorsman who freed himself the same way after trapping his hand between a boulder and a rock wall. Neither man experienced undue pain until after he had walked to safety; the American, after he had hiked for miles through the scorching southern Utah desert without water, belaying himself one-handed by rope down sandstone cliffs.

Part of the difficulty in making sense of cases like these is that what constitutes pain is not entirely clear. Pain is more likely to be expressed in grunts, shrieks, shudders, and cries than in words. Adding to its elusiveness is that pain is far from one-dimensional. It can vary by location, by duration, by intensity, and above all, by quality. It can burn, scald, sear, or sting; it can crush or press; shoot or drill; or it can quiver, flicker, throb, pulse, or beat. In other words, pain is not simply a thing that one either has or does not. It is a multifaceted, ultimately private, world.

Not only is pain complicated, it is paradoxical. Sometimes "it" can eagerly be sought out *as* a pleasure. Religious mystics have reported that the wounds they inflict on themselves are "delicious"; the agonies of their self-denials, "delightful." Even exercise junkies can be witnessed grinning back at viewers of their exercise videos, as they urge them to "feel the burn." While it is not entirely clear what these phrases mean, what appears partly to be at stake is that "pain is mine and teaches me that I exist" (Nores, 1999, 99). In other words, one of the things that attracts people to pain is the pleasure of self-certitude that it confers. To paraphrase an ancient Zen aphorism, when all things in life are false, there is one thing true, pain (Iwado, 1937, 37–39; Scarry, 1985, 4, 7, 13). This may explain the attraction of self-mutilation to alienated teenagers, or of high-risk adrenaline sports.[1]

W. I. Thomas once said that things defined as real are real in their consequences (1969, xl). So it is for pain. For pain is infinitely more than a matter of neurotransmitter function. On the contrary, "we experience pain only and entirely as we interpret it" (Morris, 1991, 2). This means that one may be severely injured yet pain-free, as in the cases of the farmer or the hiker mentioned above. Or one may suffer excruciating physical discomfort without evidence of a bodily lesion.

Joanna, a once vibrant, athletic young mother, is brought sobbing to her knees by "a ticker tape of pinpricks, an electrical storm, . . . amplified and staticky" issuing from the soles of her feet (Stein, 2007, 23). She reports that the pain worsens after she lies down, but also after she starts moving. It invariably follows exercise, but also comes with equal ferocity after a day of rest. Joanna drags herself from podiatrist to chiropractor, from psychiatrist to osteopath to find its cause, undergoing X-rays, MRIs, and blood tests, all to no avail. "I don't know how I'm going to continue like this for the next thirty years," she tearfully confesses (46). Joanna is alone with her pain.

If the experience of pain changes with the words used to frame it, pain also varies by the ways it is dramatized. For pain is not just a feeling, much less a neurological sensation; it is a culturally mediated "performance of suffering" (Illich, 1976, 133). Among other things, this suggests that there can be pain "fashions" and even pain "fashion setters" who "work" pain in such a way as to enhance their own significance and marketability, and whose displays are aped by others craving the same attention. Susan Sontag (1978) writes about how the hollow-eyed, ashen languor associated with tuberculosis (TB) was crafted into a "trope for self-assertion" in the eighteenth and nineteenth centuries, becoming a preferred body style for artists and bohemians. Period commentators argued that TB could be taken as a sign of the victim's sensitivity, their delicateness, and creativity; of their heroic refusal to swallow the "vulgarities of ordinary bourgeois life," with its rich food, warm rooms, and comfortable clothes. With TB's presumed "romantic agonies" considered a marker of glamour, Sontag says, young artists "vied" with each other to be disabled by it (26–36).[2]

Whatever the sources of expressive pain standards might be, it is well documented that the manner by which an effusive Italian enacts pain is quite different from that of the stoic Japanese; the Irishman from the cultured, pain-reactive Jew (Zborowski, 1969). We know too that wounded soldiers are far less pain-demonstrative than civilians who suffer comparable fates. Like the injured athlete who plays on for fear of "letting the team down," the bleeding soldier knows that if s/he screams in pain the morale of his or her buddies will be affected, and the battle lost. The sighs and moans indicative of chronic pain in first world nations are, according to pain experts, virtually unknown in Red China and in other places where it is simply not tolerated, or where there is no insurance to cover it (Bates et al., 1993). Contrast this with the United States where, in any year, close to one-fifth of the population reports being in chronic pain (Kolata, 1994) and where over $120 billion is lost annually to the economy because of it (Morris, 2000, 109–10). Much of this is in the form of lower back pain, which may be considered an almost signature American malady, but one virtually unreported in developing countries (Morris, 2000, 122).

Even in our era it is still not uncommon for people to speak of pain as a "challenge soliciting a response," a stage that offers them an opportunity to display virtues of patience, endurance, resignation, perseverance, and self-control, for example, to "offer it up to the Lord," or to use it as a means to burn off bad karma or, like Job, to have their faith tested. After all, as it is said, "God will never give me more than I can handle." Ivan Illich decries the fact that by transforming pain into a neurological "complaint" to be "mechanically managed," modern medicine "smothers pain's intrinsic question mark" (Illich, 1976, 143). In so doing, it lessens the opportunity for patients to address the existential questions that pain raises (149). He acknowledges that Euro-America is not alone in trying to manage pain. Every known society has a pain-alleviating arsenal that ranges from marijuana, alcohol, and coca leaves to hypnosis, massage, and poppy seeds. But he insists that "pain killing" proper—a phrase coined in 1853 by an American patent medicine dealer—is a uniquely Euro-American enterprise (151).

Illich traces the modern battle against pain back to René Descartes, whose theory still passes as orthodoxy in today's medical schools. Descartes argues that pain is a signal sent by pain receptors along nerve filaments directly to the brain in order to protect the body-machine from (further) injury. Imagine a person standing next to a fire, Descartes might say. "The flame particle jumps from the fire, touches the toe, moves up the spinal cord until a little bell goes off in the brain and says, 'Ouch. It hurts'" (Callihan, 1995, 2). This is the so-called nociceptic (i.e., pain receptor) explanation for pain. The nociceptic theory is useful when it comes to peripheral "nerve-impulse" pain, which may be considered a genetically selected blessing that promotes biological survival. However, it is far less plausible when it comes to the "deep pain" of chronic illness.

Deep pain should not be thought of so much as a sensation than as a matter of "attitude," and ultimately a product of culture. For no amount of nerve blocks, burning, or analgesics can effectively calm it. In fact, they may well aggravate it by producing secondary debilitation. David Morris relates the story of novelist Reynolds Price who underwent radiation and surgery for spinal cancer. The treatment not only rendered Price a wheelchair-bound paraplegic, it threw him into pain that "was high and all-pervading from neck to feet," a torture that would "peak in blinding storms" in the afternoon or during the onset of bad weather. Only after he underwent long sessions of biofeedback and self-hypnosis did Price's agony vanish into "scattered minutes here and there" (Morris, 2000, 116). Prior to this, imbued with the Cartesian theory that "pain means trouble," Price had unwittingly added to his own discomfort by thinking that something terrible was happening to his body each time pain would work itself past his narcotized haze. After he learned to recite the following mantra, his pain magically fled: "the harm is done. It cannot be repaired; pain signifies nothing. Begin to ignore it" (117). Joanna, the woman mentioned earlier who was tortured by foot pain, tried a similar regimen, but came away with less happy results.

It is impossible to itemize all the meanings that can intensify chronic pain. Among those enumerated by Price are fear of the future, grief at the loss of mobility, and anger over the body's betrayal. There is also the sense of being unable to control the pain when it makes its evening visits, a lack of confidence that doctors can do anything about it, and the looming specter of isolation. To these we can add three other factors to which we now turn our attention: feelings of discredit, the experience of shrinkage, and confusion.

Stigma

In *Being and Nothingness*, Jean-Paul Sartre introduces an idea that has profound implications for understanding the lived experience of illness: "the look" (*le regard*) (Sartre, 1956, 340–400). According to Sartre, the look of the other shapes the way I see and think about myself (cf. Cooley, 1902, 152). It shatters the smooth, preconscious flow of everyday life, effectively turning me into a thing. If, for instance, absorbed in traversing a crowded campus walkway I suddenly trip and fall, scattering my glasses and papers on the pavement, the immediate sensation is not one of physical pain; it is embarrassment or shame. Others are looking at me, judging me, defining me as a clod. The gaze of others leaves a stigma (from Gr. "to mark" or "brand") that colors my sense of self; it makes me acutely aware of my own body. "The Other's look," says Sartre, "fashions my body in its nakedness, causes it to be born, sculpts it, produces it as it *is*. . . . The Other holds a secret—the secret of what *I am*" (Sartre, 1956, 475, our emphasis). The role played by others in the formation of self-experience is so central to Sartre that in his play, *No Exit*, he has one of the characters conclude, "Hell is—other people!" (Sartre, 1989, 45). By merely withdrawing their gaze from us they can make us doubt our existence.

When we fall ill, the power of the other's look is magnified. We are repeatedly reminded of being damaged, disfigured, immobile, and slow. This is what happened to an already self-conscious teenager named Leila after she underwent major surgery to remove a neck tumor. Suddenly, she was no longer part of the in-crowd, those of her classmates who took pleasure in judging outsiders. She *was* the outsider (Stein, 2007, 122–23, 139–45).

When normals hold the door at the grocery store or help you down the stairs, when the child gawks, or the co-worker asks, "Is everything all right?" your body unveils itself as broken. You are marked with discredit and begin to see yourself as "not quite human" (Goffman, 1963). Take the case of a woman who has had her colon removed and who now wears a sickly-sweet scented colostomy bag to collect the contents of her bowels.

> I feel so embarrassed by this—this thing. It seems so unnatural, so dirty. I can't get used to the smell [of] it. I'm scared of soiling myself. Then I'd be so ashamed I couldn't look at anyone else. . . . Who would want a wife like this? How can I go out and . . . look people in the eyes and tell them the truth? Once I do, who would want to develop a friendship, I mean a close one? How can I even consider showing my body to someone else, having sex? . . . I feel terrible, like a monster. (Kleinman, 1988, 63)

This woman's shame prompts her either to conceal her condition or to avoid potentially degrading situations altogether: concerts, athletic events, or personal dates. She flees into the security of isolation.

Where complete withdrawal is impossible, which is almost always true, the ill employ different tactics so as not to draw untoward attention to themselves. One is to not take issue with boorish comments from normals about people like themselves: AIDS victims, cancer sufferers, or addicts. Goffman tells of ex-mental patients who are reluctant to engage in barbed exchanges with spouses or friends for fear that any show of emotion might be interpreted as confirmation of their enduring defect (Goffman, 1963, 13).

Another ploy is to hide one's blemish with an artificial device or a concealing garment. Leila, the girl described above, disfigured by the red surgical scar on her neck, tells her doctor about "really weird dreams about masks and veils. After school, I go from drugstore to drugstore, searching for makeup to cover myself, to make my neck secret" (Stein, 2007, 139).

Still another tactic is to undergo "repair work" on a misshapen body part. In addition to surgeries there is, as discussed in chapter 3, a growing industry of cosmetic pharmacology that can be used to present one's self more artfully in public: to be more serene and less combative, a better "team player," "more fun to be around." We will have more to say about repair work in the next chapter.

Goffman identifies a fourth tactic, which he calls "painful mimicry" of the bodily comportment of normals. In 1988, Republican presidential candidate Robert Dole attempted to conceal his World War II injury by clutching a pen to his chest, making it appear as if his arm and hand were working normally. Democratic president Franklin Roosevelt successfully hid his inability to stand by deploying pre-placed podium props and supports. Among the latter were aides strategically positioned to hoist him from limousines and railroad cars.

This brings us to a fifth measure, using normals to "cover" for them. What we mean by this are wives who punch phone numbers for their Parkinson's stricken husbands, or spouses who serve as each others' ears, eyes, or mouths. Today, it is increasingly common to witness young, athletic normals leading amputees down ski slopes by cables and sleds, or carrying them up on their backs to afford them the "full wilderness experience." While all this is intended to help an ill person "pass" as normal, accepting help from others does not come without a price. It can underscore one's neediness and negatively impact their esteem. This is why victims can sometimes be seen to angrily insist, "I don't need you . . . I can do it myself!" That they often cannot only amplifies their compromised status.

In addition to offering physical aid, loved ones and companions can also be relied upon for "elaborate lies," as Goffman calls them: stories about why s/he is once again late for work, cannot come to the party, or will not be able to go on the weekend retreat. But this too is not without its problems. After all, who can I trust with my degrading secret without fear of ridicule? Even helpful gestures may be viewed by victims through the lens of their own stigma: "they are only being nice because of my illness."[3]

Everything we have just enumerated is amplified when pain, nausea, dizziness, or tiredness are considered by significant others to be "unreal" or "only in your head." This is particularly prevalent with persistent somatoform conditions like chronic fatigue or debilitating, yet phantom pains that are not traceable to a physiological cause. Here are the words of a woman suffering from chronic back pain following a car crash:

> I have an "invisible" disability. Judging from the surprised reactions when I explain my problem ("but you look fine"), I appear healthy, vigorous and energetic. [Yet] I cannot go for both dinner and the movie, because it involves extended sitting. . . . Travel and airports pose obstacles, and have sometimes ended in unpleasant incidents. I am unable to lift my luggage from my rolling cart to the x-ray security trolley. Some airport staff have refused to assist. I have been asked mockingly, *"Are you an invalid?"* (Freund et al., 2003, 148)

This woman's plight is doubly problematic. Not only is she discredited by her impairment, but given that its source is invisible, she is also at risk of being judged disobedient or even crazy. This label carries its own sanctions that we need not address here.

In sum, each of us yearns to nurture and protect what George Herbert Mead once described as "our most precious part," our sense of worth. But illness threatens our validity as human beings. It renders us invalid. This brings us to consideration of still another set of impression management maneuvers: bodily jujitsu, turning illness back on itself to enhance one's esteem. One form of this is to use one's condition as a "hook" (Goffman's term) on which to hang their failures after the fact, or as a disclaimer to alert others of an imminent mishap: "I really am a talented . . . but I've been ill and out of practice; so don't expect too much." Another is to count the illness as a blessing, as in "it's the best thing that ever happened to me. Before this, I took things for granted." A third tack is to "come out," to publicly broadcast one's illness instead of concealing it (Lerner, 2006). When celebrity patients such as basketball star Magic Johnson (HIV+), Tour de France champion Lance Armstrong (testicular cancer), or award-winning entertainers like Christopher Reeve (quadriplegia) and Michael J. Fox (Parkinson's) turned their private sufferings into major media events, this had two consequences. First, they were regaled as heroes. Second, by putting a "face" on the illness, their disclosures helped normalize those who, until recently, had been discredited for having comparable conditions.

Shrinkage

Shrinking Space

Our bodies display their own kinesthetic wisdom, their *praktognosia*, as Maurice Merleau-Ponty calls it. By this he means an ability to seamlessly and prereflectively maneuver through, handle, and orient itself within lived space (Merleau-Ponty, 1962, 140–41). Lived space is not to be confused with geometric space, a three-dimensional coordinate system of length, height, and depth within which interchangeable objects reside. It is, rather, the familiar horizon or setting produced by our customary ways of walking, reaching, manipulating, and using various things (102). These ways of navigating, of *living* space, serve to shape who we understand ourselves to be. For example, by embodying the concrete activity of a college professor—walking to the office, preparing manuscripts on the computer, lecturing in front of class—I understand myself *as* a professor. I *am* what I *do* (Heidegger, 1962, 283).

When I am healthy, my body stretches "ex-statically" into lived space, beyond the limits of my skin. The lived-body and the world "intersect and engage each other like gears" as I climb stairs, open doors, and sit at the desk (Merleau-Ponty, 1962, xx). It is in those moments that I feel "I can" (137). When the lived-body is ill, on the other hand, this disposition shifts dramatically to "I can't" (cf. Young, 1990). Now the world no longer gives itself as an expansive horizon of possibilities into which I can pass. Instead, the stairs look *insurmountable,* the door is *too heavy,* and sitting *is painful.* The boundaries of my world begin to collapse (Toombs, 1992, 66–68, 82–83).

Pain plays a central role in shrinkage, as suggested by the metaphors used to describe it. Pain is said to "tighten" my facial expression into a grimace or to "contort" my muscles. My sciatic nerve "pinches," my stomach "cramps," my chest feels like it's "clamped" in a vise. Following a car accident, one woman characterized her pain as "a big lump—red and hot—of muscles, nerves, and tendons bunched together in my upper back. . . . The pain feels like it comes from tightness, tension. It already limits my . . . activities" (Kleinman, 1988, 90). As she monitors and manages her pain, this woman's life shrivels. The freedoms she once took for granted—strolling the sidewalk, handling the mail, typing, anticipating a vacation—begin to break down. Pain insinuates itself so intimately into her affairs that it becomes who she is: "It controls me . . . stops me." Now every decision must be put off until *she* can "control it" (Kleinman, 1988, 91).

A diabetic concurs. First he "lost his birthday" while in the hospital being diagnosed, then his favorite food. He "lost his fantasy of good health," followed in rapid succession by his vision, his job, and his ability to walk, all of which took away his independence. Then he lost his sexual virility and with it, his wife's affection, followed by that of his children and later his mother, whom he could no longer care for. Finally, after he began to lose body parts, amputated to halt the spread of infection, he discouraged his friends from visiting. In the end his life had shrunk to the dimensions of maintaining proper glucose levels (Stein, 2007, 121; cf. Kleinman, 1988, 37).

The sense of shrinkage can be aggravated by how living spaces are architecturally constructed to meet the specifications of normals. Thus, the flight of granite stairs at the courthouse entrance that seems so beautifully striking to normals is experienced by the wheelchaired citizen as just one more hindrance to mobility. "Chairs without arms to push . . . up from; unpadded seats which . . . produced sores; . . . toilets without handrails. . . ;

surfaces too slippery to walk on; staircases without banisters; buildings without ramps, . . . ; every curbstone a precipice": the very things blithely unnoticed by normals, turn space into a nightmare of blockades for the ill (Freund et al., 2003, 161). Because of these architectural impediments, those who are impaired become effectively disabled, not by the physical wound or injury as such, but by the institutionalized failure to accommodate their needs. Imagine yourself born, full-sighted, into a world constructed for the blind, with Braille libraries, no incandescent lighting, and movement regulated entirely by sounds: you too would be disabled (161).

Because the lifeworld is shared with others, shrinkage has social impacts. When the world becomes unmanageable and threatening, the ill begin to withdraw from it. This is not only because being engaged requires normal mobility and functioning—for example, urinary continence, the ability to feed oneself, and to hear—but also because of others' condescending gestures, stares, and thoughtless queries. At the same time, because they are marked by the difference conferred upon them by illness—a difference that can remind normals of their own precariousness—the presence of the ill in classrooms, on the job, or at the dance can make normals decidedly uncomfortable. "What should I say?" "Should I offer help?" "If I pretend not to notice, will they be insulted?" The result is mutual avoidance and isolation (Stein, 2007). Here is the confession of one person: "I feel . . . sad about being ill. . . . I feel headaches, dizziness, don't like to talk, take no pleasure in things. My head and eyes are swollen. My hair is falling out. My thinking has slowed down. *[The] symptoms are worse when I am with others, better when I am alone*" (Kleinman, 1988, 108, our emphasis).

But things are not always as simple as this. Occasionally, because of marriage vows, the duties of parenthood, or the need to care for one's own mother and father, the shrinkage endemic to illness can become contagious. Its deadening viscosity can contaminate helpers. The world of family and friends can be swallowed by the narrow parameters of the victim. Here, a retired lawyer describes the impact of his wife's Alzheimer's on him and his children.

Our children come and they cry. And I cry. We reminisce about
old times. We try to recall what Anna was like before. . . . But I
can see it wears them out just being here for a day or two.
They've got their own troubles. I can't ask them to help out any
more than they do already. Me? It's made a different person
out of me. I expect you wouldn't have recognized me if you
had met me ten years ago. I feel at least ten years older than I
am. I'm afraid of what will happen if I go first. I haven't had a
half hour free of worry and hurt for ten years. This illness
didn't just destroy Anna's mind, it has killed something in me,
in the family, too. If anyone asks about Alzheimer's, tell them
it is a disease of the whole family. (Kleinman, 1988, 183)

The interplay between the management of symptoms and social
isolation creates a negative feedback loop. Each insidiously feeds
off the other, making them worse than either alone might otherwise be. My life retreats back to the boundaries of my corporeal-
ity, back to my *Körper*, to the corpse. I become "dead," dead in
life, depressed.

Thomas Fuchs, drawing on the work of Merleau-Ponty, proposes that depression be regarded as a form of "bodily restric-
tion" (Fuchs, 2005, 99; 2003, 237), a "freezing or rigidity of the
lived-body" that can localize in a specific organ: "a feeling of an
armor [around] the chest, of a lump in the throat, pressure in the
head." Or depression can be experienced as a diffuse anxiety
permeating one's entire flesh. (The German *Angst* and the Latin
anguistiae both point to a narrowing or restricting [Fuchs, 2003,
237]). As the lived-body contracts to its own skin, the everyday
world loses its felt richness and familiarity. Visual and audio
cues are abstracted from a larger context and show up as simple
sensations denuded of meaning. Otherwise compelling or tragic
life events are experienced with emotional flatness and indifference.

In *The Stranger*, Albert Camus' central character, Meursault,
is pictured this way. Following his mother's funeral, it occurs to
him "that somehow I'd gotten through another Sunday, that
Mother now was buried, and tomorrow I'd be going back to
work as usual. Really, nothing in my life had changed" (Camus,
1946, 30). When asked by his girlfriend whether he loves her, he

answers, "the question mean[s] nothing or next to nothing" (52). Even his murder of a complete stranger and subsequent death sentence leave Mersault unfazed and bored. He confesses that he has "lost the habit of noting feelings. . . . Nothing, nothing had [any] significance" (80, 152). Fuchs would explain Meursault's depression as a "loss of body resonance" wherein one is rendered incapable of "feeling themselves into the world" (Fuchs, 2005, 100).

Expansive, unfettered connectedness to the world enables the gestures of colleagues, friends, and family to enter us as meaningful acts, not merely as mechanical operations. Upturned mouths become smiles; moisture on the cheek, tears; an empty palm held out to us, a sign of peace. By the same token, the inability to feel into the world forecloses any possibility of emotional connection to others. Instead, they present themselves as "little robot[s]," to quote Meursault. Fuchs provides powerful testimony of this from one of his patients who is so shutdown that he imagines himself already dead.

> Someone who resembled my wife, was walking beside me, and my friend visited me. . . . Everything was as it would be normally. The figure representing my wife constantly reminded me of what I had failed to do for her. . . . What looks like normal life is not. I found myself on the other side. And now I realized what the cause had been. . . . I had died, but God had removed this event from my consciousness. . . . A harsher punishment could hardly be imagined. Without being aware of having died, you are in a hell that resembles in all details the world you had lived in, and thus God lets you see and feel that you have made nothing of your life. (Fuchs, 2003, 238–39)

Fuchs cites other patients who report having no feelings at all. One sixty-five-year-old woman "maintained that her body, her stomach and bowels had been contracted so long that there was no hollow space left. Her whole body, she said, was dried out, nothing moved anymore; she sensed neither heat nor cold. She could not even die, for everything was already dry and dead" (Fuchs, n.d., 8).

Psychiatrist Marie Åsberg expands on Fuchs's account of bodily shrinkage in her portrayal of "The Exhaustion Funnel."

According to Åsberg, because of the fatigue and indifference that accompany depression, we begin to give up nonessential, normally enjoyable activities like gardening, exercise, going to movies, long talks with friends, and listening to music. That is to say, there is a narrowing or "funneling" of our existence down to essentials. Life closes in on us; we stop doing the things that once nourished and enriched us, leaving only work or other stressors that continue to deplete our emotional resources. The narrower the funnel becomes, the easier it is to be drawn into the hollowed-out state of having but one choice, either to live or to die (Williams et al., 2007, 28–29).

Shrinking Time

Human being not only has a spatial dimension. As we saw in chapter 3, it is also temporal. To quote Richard Zaner, we "embody rhythmically and episodically" (Zaner, 1981, 58). We do this in two ways. First, the body's organs have their own tempos. The heart has its pulse; the sleep center of the brain, its circadian cycle; the digestive system, its metabolic rate; and so on. These can go on without "me" ever being aware of them. The second way by which we are temporally embodied arises from the fact that we are more than just things, more than merely organ systems (*Körper*). We are persons, and personhood implies a capacity to act: to anticipate what-is-to-come (the future) relative to what is now (the present) and to what once was (the past). This is what is meant by *lived* time (58). In contrast to the pace of biological rhythms, which are largely veiled to me, by means of purposive action the embodied *I* unfolds into the world; who *I* am as a person becomes manifestly real.

Lived time in this sense has its own rhythm and beat. At one moment I act with tense-faced urgency; at another, with a cool, relaxed, bearing. Normally, I "go with the flow," moving easily with changing circumstances. When I am maimed or ill, however, the body executes my will painfully, poorly, or not at all. When this occurs, lived time, time *as it is for me*, shrinks (Toombs, 1992, 68–70). Its once open vista of future hopes and dreams collapses into a single temporal dimension: the present. Caught up in the immediacy of managing pain and discomfort, just to think about the future becomes exhausting. One woman writes, "[M]y health is too uncertain. I cannot do too much. I think only of my [pain], not of the future" (Kleinman, 1988, 107). Nor, she adds, "of the past." The lived past with its remembered images of vitality and independence closes off. The remaining memories are stripped of their emotional valence and begin showing up in an alien and abstract way as the experiences of someone else. This too is a hallmark of depression: a state wherein any dimension but the present and its agonies is inconceivable. "It has always been like this, and it will stay the same for ever—all reminiscence or hope different from that is deception" (Fuchs, n.d., 10).

Illness profoundly impacts one's capacity to live in accordance with the demands of modern time where a premium is placed on productive efficiency and, above all, on speed. Added to this is the fact that the ill who are also uninsured often cannot "afford" to take a day off to recuperate, much less a week or a month, when symptoms flare up. This, naturally, makes it difficult for them to recover. "The trouble is," says one woman, "I never fully recuperated. *I didn't have the time.* I had to get back to work or I would have lost the only job I could find" (Kleinman, 1988, 112, our emphasis). She goes on describe her fear that she will never get better. But insofar as the anticipated shame of being fired is even worse, she redoubles her effort to keep up with the relentless ticking of the office clock, aggravating her already compromised condition: "My overachiever pattern that got me sick [in the first place] was still in gear. I felt ashamed of being sick, of falling behind, and needed to push myself." She finally surrenders to the necessity that "I need to let myself be sick, not push myself to be healthy" (113).

Confusion

Ordinarily, death is interpreted as a biological accident or as mishap that occurs in slow stages and is always far off in the distance. It is an event from which we are disengaged, something that happens to the sick, the elderly, or the foolish—not to me.

Leo Tolstoy's *The Death of Ivan Ilych* provides a classic rendition of this mindset. At Ilych's funeral his friend, Peter Ivanovich, is momentarily awakened to the terrifying reality of his own inevitable death. But then he immediately pushes the specter away as irrational and morbid. "After which . . . Peter Ivanovich felt reassured, and began to ask with interest about the details of Ivan Ilych's death, as though death was an accident natural to Ivan Ilych but certainly not to himself" (Tolstoy, 1960, 102).

To the chronically ill, this kind of detachment is difficult. One is constantly reminded of death, not as an anonymous biological event, but as the ultimate existential given, as *mine*, as something that happens to *me*. A young man dying of cancer describes the absurd horror of it:

> Do you know, can you imagine what it—it feels like to make that statement and know that it is true for you, that you are dying. . . . All that nonsense that's written [e.g., by Elisabeth Kübler-Ross] about stages of dying, as if there were complete transitions—rooms that you enter, walk through, then leave behind for good. What rot. The anger, the shock, the unbelievableness, the grief—they are part of each day. . . . I don't want to die. I'm only thirty-three; I've got my whole life to live. I can't be cut off now. It isn't just. Why me? Why now? (Kleinman, 1988, 147)

Added to these questions are others: Why this? What will happen? Will I ever be able to walk again? To read? To see my grandchildren? Does the pain only get worse? Will I be able to stand it? What will happen to my spouse and all those dreams we shared? What was the point of all the energy and time I invested at work?

We don't just want to know the meaning of our condition, its medical diagnosis; we want to grasp its meaning*fulness*. Unable to put into words the larger significance of our deaths, we are thrown into confusion, angered by the affront to our dignity.

To be sure, religions provide stock consolations: it's your karma, for example, the inevitable consequence of choices you made long ago. Or it's the divine justice of a God who has His reasons. It is dumb fate, or the product of our overattachment to unreal things. While all of these can be traced to the personal agonies undergone by the prophets who first announced them, they are now, too often, bowdlerized clichés. They may be fit to address death in general at memorial services, but they are far less convincing when it comes to my own personal demise, my own suffering.

Our public involvements and private concerns give us a sense of cohesion and purpose. We lose ourselves in them. And when we do so, we forget about our ultimate contingency and the precariousness of life. The job and travel, the vitamin regimens, the proper diet and exercise, the "soft addictions" to gadgets and Facebook gossip, and the voyeuristic glutting of ourselves with pornography, sports, and news updates: all of these permit "a constant tranquilization about death." This includes the deaths of other people, which begin to be seen, as Ilych's is for Peter Ivanovich, as a "social inconvenience." The deaths of others come to be felt as displaying a lack of consideration for me, "if not . . . a downright tactlessness," something against which we have a right to be protected (Heidegger, 1962, 297–98).

We can be rudely yanked out of this benumbed state of self-absorption by crises, particularly when they are unlooked for. Illness is an example that, if serious enough, can plunge us into the depths of *Angst* (anxiety). For philosophers like Heidegger, *Angst* is not the same thing as fear, for fear requires an object. Fear is always about something: flying, germs, the upcoming exam, terrorism, and the like. In contrast, angst concerns nothing at all, nothing. It is the unsettling realization that my heretofore neatly arranged existence is penetrated to its very core by an abyss. "Anxiety," says Heidegger, "reveals the nothing. . . . [It] leaves us hanging because it induces the slipping away of *beings as a whole*" (Heidegger, 1977c, 103). We cannot point to the object that causes anxiety because there is nothing to point to. We are, simply, anxious in the face of nothing.

Medical professionals are largely helpless when it comes to this kind of deep anxiety (Stein, 2007). After all, their field of expertise is the *Körper*, the seeable workings and malfunctions of our biology. They passionately search for answers, for ways to alleviate the pains, cure the disease, but death is not a disease; it has no answer. It is precisely the powerlessness of medicine in the face of death that drives Ivan Ilych mad. His doctors try to console Ilych with news that his fevered exhaustion and nausea are due to a ruptured appendix or a floating kidney. But Ilych knows better.

> It's not a question of appendix or kidney, but of life and . . . death. Yes, life was there and now it is going, going and I cannot stop it. Yes. Why deceive myself? . . . There was light and now there is darkness. I was here and now I'm going there! Where? . . . When I'm not, what will there be? There will be nothing. Then where shall I be when I am no more? Can this be dying? No, I don't want to! . . . It is impossible that all men have been doomed to suffer this awful horror. (Tolstoy, 1960, 130)

Ilych's doctors cannot find death, cannot take it from him. This is because death is not an object to be surgically removed as if it were a tumor or an infection. One's own death is a fundamental structure of being human. And just as no one can live my life, "no one can take [my own death] away from [me]" (Heidegger, 1962, 284). To alleviate himself from the burden of this truth, Ilych tries to tell his wife about "something terrible" he now knows about himself, something "more important than anything before in his life." However, she soon becomes bored with his story. When her daughter arrives with the baby, she sighs, and they scurry out the door to go shopping.

Irvin Yalom points out that the helplessness and despair that accompany death anxiety is so profound that most of us are driven to repress it and then unconsciously to transfer it onto a convenient object, a "problem" that we can solve. It becomes my agoraphobia, for example; my fear of crowds; or even better, my fear of an enemy "out there" that I can battle. And while the antidepressants, the yoga classes, the cognitive behavioral training, and wars are annoying and expensive, they nonetheless make life manageable. Like the curtains that Ivan Ilych and his wife hang on the parlor windows to keep out the black Russian winter just prior to the accident that will thrust Ilych permanently into night, these objective worries keep me from having to deal with my own yawning emptiness. Heidegger agrees; the drift and "tug" (*Zug*) of my daily worries "make things easy for me." They allow me to "take my ease" (Heidegger, 2001b, 81). "In caring [about them], life sequesters itself off from itself" (80). Worried tonight to the point of insomnia about tomorrow, or ruing the fool I made of myself yesterday, I am not right here, accepting that my factical life "has its time" (103).

Chronic illness makes repression of death anxiety virtually impossible. The visceral awareness of my inevitable end is woven into the fabric of my routines. The humiliations attendant to my impairments or those inflicted on me by thoughtless normals, coupled with my pain-induced diminishment serve as unrelenting reminders of my fate. But—and this is crucial—this same awareness also holds seeds of personal growth into wholeness, which is to say, into health, if not into a cure. It can open us to the possibility of being authentic. This is described by Heidegger as a condition of "self-gathering" out of our scattered dispersion in the opinions and expectations of "the they" (*das Man*), of anyone and everyone. It has the power to awaken us from the slumber of shallow preoccupations to the preciousness and fragility of life. One begins to see things more clearly and vividly.

From his years of work with terminally ill cancer patients, Yalom can cite many cases of conversion to authenticity. Here are the words of Senator Richard Neuberger, composed shortly before his death from cancer:

> A change came over me which I believe is irreversible. Questions of prestige, of political success, of financial status, became all at once unimportant. In those first hours when I realized I had cancer, I never thought of my seat in the Senate, of my bank account, or of the destiny of the free world. . . . My wife and I have not had a quarrel since my illness was diagnosed. I used to scold her about squeezing the toothpaste from the top instead of the bottom, about not catering sufficiently to my fussy appetite, about making up guest lists without consulting me, about spending too much on clothes.

Now I am either unaware of such matters, or they seem irrelevant. . . . In their stead has come a new appreciation of
things I once took for granted—eating lunch with a friend,
scratching Muffet's ears and listening for his purrs, the company of my wife, reading a book or magazine in the quiet
cone of my bed lamp at night, raiding the refrigerator for a
glass of orange juice or coffee cake. For the first time I think
I actually am savoring life. . . . I realize, finally, what I spoiled
for myself . . . by false pride, synthetic values, and fancied
slights. (Yalom, 1980, 35; for other examples, see Levine,
1989)

For Neuberger and others like him, once death has visited,
life's priorities rearrange themselves. Postponing living until
one gets the degree, earns their tenure, the kids graduate, or
until the "golden years" of retirement becomes unacceptable:
"Trivialities are trivialized." What they, the anonymous other,
think becomes irrelevant, fears of rejection vanish, and risk-
taking seems reasonable. There is an enhanced sense of urgency, of joy in small things, and of gratitude for the gift of
life. Kathy, a victim of kidney failure that nearly killed her, reports that

I am [now] infatuated with life. Look at the beauty in the sky!
It's gorgeously blue! I go into a flower garden and every flower
takes on such fabulous colors and I am dazzled. . . . One thing
I do know, had I remained my first Kathy, I would have played
away my whole life, and I would never have known what the
real joy of living was all about. I had to face death eyeball to
eyeball before I could live. I had to die in order to live. (Yalom,
1980, 38)

Death-inspired existential wisdom can impart courage, resolute-
ness, and thankfulness. It can nourish one's capacity for compassion and enable us to forgive. In short, it can expose who we
really are beneath our self-concerned dramas. All attempts to
control and/or displace death anxiety fall away. Life reveals itself in a fresh new way, infinitely valuable, uncertain, and mysterious.

Notes

1. The reader hardly needs to be reminded that passion or suffering (from which we get the word "patient") is a fundamental component of love. Widely considered one of the most highly valued conditions, love's patron is pictured as a wounding arrow-armed boy, Amor (Eros = Cupid).

2. The reader may recall, more recently, the exploding popularity of multiple personality disorder among middle-class women in America during the late 1980s. See chapter 4, note 13.

3. There is one tactic Goffman cautions against. Do not, he warns, become a "stigma clown." Never try to put normals at ease by making fun of your illness. While the intention in doing so may be to deflect the critical gaze of the other, it can backfire. It may make normals even more uncomfortable, more ready to avoid you. But why, we might ask, must it be the victim's responsibility to put normals at ease? Goffman's reply: It is just one more Kafkaesque "social fact" of lived illness, to be ignored at your own peril. After all, things could be worse; you could be "put away," permanently exiled to a ghetto built for stigmatics: an assisted care unit or a nursing home.

7

Medicine and Phenomenology

Being-Toward-Death

The human being, says Heidegger, is that being whose being is an issue for it (Heidegger, 1962, 32). This is reflected by the care I embody toward things, the way I fret about them and exhibit concern (*Besorgen*). As a teacher, I worry about the student who struggles in class. As a professor, I hold extended office hours because I care about my self-interpretation as a responsible person. As a university employee, I brood about its financial condition. These ways of living, of caring, of being "there" in academia are but one dimension in a wider web of social relations, practices, and apprehensions, the totality of which we can call, simply, "the world."

In everyday life, my anger, discouragement, or happiness are always directed toward one concern or another.[1] I am upset *about* my brother's divorce, happy *that* I got a raise at work, angry *over* a colleague's betrayal, and distressed *by* reports of global warming. Above all, I worry about the generalized other, them (*das Man*), what they think about me, and adjust my behaviors and values accordingly: "[I] take pleasure as *they* take pleasure; see, read, and judge . . . literature and art as *they* do; . . . shrink back from the 'great mass' as *they* shrink back; . . . find 'shocking' what *they* find shocking" (Heidegger, 1962, 164). For all my well-crafted, self-advertised singularity, in other words, I am actually a "they-self" (*Man-selbst*).

As we saw in the last chapter, my worldly cares provide comfort and security. They allow me to avoid dealing with "my own-most possibility," as Heidegger phrases it: my own death. Ernest Becker agrees; the story of our being-in-the-world, he says, is at heart a narrative of death denial (Becker, 1973; Becker, 1975). He goes on to provide a kaleidoscope of preoccupations by which humans "escape evil."[2]

First and foremost, says Becker, there is involvement in salvation religions that promise eternal life in the hereafter to devotees: door-to-door evangelizing, the attendance of services at mosque or synagogue, praying, and tithing. Next in order comes the accumulation of possessions: cowrie shells, gold nuggets, paper deeds, stock certificates, and "life insurance" policies. Then there is marriage through which a man can expend his seed and extend his existence. Another is participation in massive public works projects, especially crusades to "save the world" from death's supposed carriers: Nazis, Commies, capitalist "running dogs," swarthy-skinned Jews, Nips, and Huns. Last are efforts to separate ourselves from unclean people and things—from alien music and images, strange foods and intoxicants—either by erecting fences and moats between us and them, or by fastidiously policing our bodies' orifices (J. Aho, 2002). By means of these "well-adjusted neuroses," as Becker calls them, people convince themselves that their "thrown-ness" into the infinity of a silent universe has ultimate meaning or, as Becker would phrase it, that we are "heroic" (Becker, 1973, 178–79). The "rub," he continues, is that while these and related tactics allow us to pretend that we have overcome death, like Freud's return of the repressed, they boomerang back to become sources of our own "destructive demonism."

Becker's academic career began at the Upstate Medical Center in Syracuse, New York. It is therefore a bit ironic that, with the exception of psychotherapy, his itemization of death denials fails to mention the healing arts. For outside of religion, historically no other enterprise plays such a seminal role in dealing with the scourges of flesh than this. In our era, it is neither primarily through faith, money, holy war, offspring, nor morality that more and better life is conferred. It is through the gifts bestowed to us by scientific biomedicine.

Enframing Our Lack

Sin

During the European age of faith (ca. 400 CE to ca. 1500 CE) private and public life were both circumscribed by the all-encompassing "sacred canopy" of the medieval church (Berger, 1969). The pace of community life was regulated according to the *ordo*, the sacred calendar which, as we observed in chapter three, consisted of at least 120 holy days during which pious folk were to abstain from ungodly activities. Each day was devoted to celebrating a particular saint, martyr, holy virgin, or, in the case of major feasts, Christ Himself. As for individual believers, every passage in their short stay on earth was mediated by one or more of the seven sacraments, so numbered after the five planets visible to the eye, plus moon and sun: "On earth as it is in heaven." Of these sacraments the most important was penance, whose allopathic unguents, detailed in chapter 5, were said to be administered by "spiritual physicians."

Long before sacramental penance was devised, Christians already shared a conviction that the earth and its denizens were fallen. What penance effected was the interiorizing of contempt. Terror of the world "out there" was deflected inward, assuming the form of wicked cravings and devilish thoughts. The faithful began experiencing themselves as "demons clothed in flesh" or as "sewers of iniquity" (J. Aho, 2005, 24–25). In other words, their sense of "existential lack," as David Loy phrases it, was enframed in the language of individual depravity: sin (Loy, 2002).

The Protestant Reformation (ca. 1550) permanently shattered the medieval world. First, as we saw earlier, it prompted the introduction of clocks into the everyday lives of the laity, replacing the ordo of sacred time with a profane linear continuum of minutes, days, and hours. Of equal importance, it put an end to the entire Roman Catholic system of jurisprudence. Gone was auricular confession, and with it the priestly power to heal sick souls through utterance of the magical words, *Ego te absolvo* ("I absolve you"). Gone too was Purgatory (a postmortem status halfway between heaven and earth where souls could be purged of those sins not yet absolved), the practice of indulgences (by which for a fee one could shorten their sentence in Purgatory), and the ecclesiastical *thesaurus* (a treasury of credits accumulated by saints that could be applied to the moral ledgers of the faithful).

Protestantism did not diminish the sense of mankind's depravity. On the contrary, it enhanced it. John Calvin went so far as to assert that while infants just out of the womb have yet to produce the fruits of iniquity, their "whole nature is . . . a seed of sin and therefore cannot but be odious and abominable to God" (Calvin, 1956, 26). What Protestantism accomplished, in fact, was the elimination of what up to then had been the technologies essential to be delivered from it. Henceforth, each believer would be thrown back on their own resources to be redeemed. Max Weber cites this as the motive behind the obsessive pursuit of money by the early Protestant sectarians (Weber, 1958). By means of riches they could convince themselves that, as the elected, at least *they* were saved.

A second tactic favored by Protestants to relieve them of death-anxiety was biomedicine; that is, the reframing of their sense of lack in biomedical terms, as a sickness rather than a sin. Now, the cure for what ailed them would no longer be found in the introspective contemplation of the soul, but in visual inspection of the body.

Sickness

We don't have to reiterate the roles played by Harvey, Bernard, Pasteur, and the like in the evolution of medical science. All that needs to be emphasized here is that with it, mankind's hopes for well-being were transferred out of the hands of priests into those of the doctor. True, it would still be primarily a white male figure who monopolized access to more and better life. True too that biomedicine as we know it today would remain in a state of childhood for at least a century and half after 1550, and that it would not succeed in freeing itself from camp followers like barbers, veterinarians, and patent medicine dealers until some time after this. However, by 1650 the seeds for the sprawling electronically equipped medical campus of our time had been planted. Ordinary life was on the way to becoming medicalized. The result today is a proliferation of physicians, counselors, therapists, trainers, and nutritionists. And following in their wake has come an avalanche of maladies. This is so much the case that one critic laughingly writes of the "disease of the month." Like the sorcerer's apprentice, he says, "the faster they try to sweep away . . . illness, the longer and faster they must keep on sweeping" (Morris, 2000, 65). In place of the confessional biographies of the late Middle Ages authored by luminaries like Francisco Petrarch or Margery Kempe, we now have an entirely new literary genre: the medical "pathography" (63). Ivan Illich summarizes the contemporary situation this way:

> From Stockholm to Wichita the towers of the medical center impress on the landscape the promise of a conspicuous final embrace. For rich and poor, life is turned into a pilgrimage through check-ups and clinics back to the ward where it started. . . . Life is reduced to a "span," . . . which, for better or worse, must be institutionally planned and shaped. . . . [It] is brought into existence with the prenatal check-up, . . . and it will end with the mark on a chart ordering resuscitation suspended. Between delivery and termination this bundle of biomedical care fits best into a city that is built like a mechanical womb. (Illich, 1976, 79)

The Medicalization of Existence

Beauty

Human beings have always been less than completely content with their natural endowments and have, like artists at the easels of their own bodies, sought to improve on them by painting, adorning, and mutilating their flesh: piercing, tattooing, foot binding, applying lead makeups and mercury-based vermillion rouges, starving themselves, and gorging (Donohoe, 2006). Most often, the artists in question have been female. What is new is aesthetic *surgery*, the quest for beauty showing up in the modern lifeworld as a medical procedure. One of the first examples of this was the Italian physician, Gaspare Tagliacozzi, who in 1597 authored an illustrated guide for performing nose jobs on, among others, victims of syphilis—this, by using skin flaps from the patients' upper arms as nasal prostheses (Kuczynski, 2006). The church protested Tagliacozzi's operation, insisting that the loss of one's nose was a just penance for sexual venery. But it was all to no avail. Today aesthetic surgeries range from relatively minor, if painful, Botox and Restylane treatments, skin abrasions, braces and porcelain-teeth veneers, hair implants or depilation, and freckle-removal to more dangerous, occasionally deadly, maneuvers: liposuction; calf, chin, penis, and breast implants; vaginoplasty; and gastric stapling. There are also scalp lifts, eyelid lifts, "foot-face lifts," "smile lifts," "butt lifts," and "labia lifts."

Alex Kuczynski bases her account of this emerging industry on ten years of field research as a self-confessed addict-observer. This included her attendance at "surgery safaris" where groups of "beauty nuns" would pilgrimage en masse to a selected physician. Elsewhere, others have reported about clinic-sponsored "Botox nights" and on in-home Botox parties, modeled after Tupperware sales campaigns.

Using intentionality as a marker of difference, Kuczynski distinguishes between plastic surgery proper versus cutting and burning for "cosmetic" ends. The purpose of the first is to repair accident injuries, war wounds, or birth defects, which is to say, bona fide diseases. The second serve merely to aggrandize the patient's vanity. However, her effort to bring moral order to an institution in which Americans invest billions of dollars annually fails in the end. The line between the two blurs, and finally disappears. There are two reasons for this. One is that the mental anguish that comes from failing to live up to standards of attractiveness, solemnly decreed by movie stars—many of whom have undergone "treatment" themselves—has been medicalized. Thin calves, sunken pectorals, shortness, tiny breasts, warts, moles, bunions, and baldness are no longer fates to be suffered with dignity; they are "diseases" to be fought with vigor. To use a different metaphor, "beauty is a commodity to be acquired by the many rather than a cosmic gift mysteriously granted to the elect" (Mead, 2006, 90). A second reason is that popular "makeover reality" TV shows have so normalized the operations that they have become composites in the kit bag of ordinary possibilities and needs. As the advertisement says, "Everybody does it. Isn't it time for you . . . ?" Everybody: Heidegger's *das Man*, the anonymous "they." With this declaration, a whole new field of concern is baptized: enhancement medicine.

Proponents of enhancement medicine argue that insofar as every human being is, relative to one standard or another, abnormal—whether in terms of foot speed, IQ, blue-eyed blondness, masculinity, or conviviality—they are therefore "disabled" and deserving of treatment (Wolbring, 2006). Thus far, implementation of this ambition has come up against the hard realities of insurance company suspicions and/or the limits of most people's checkbooks. However, fertility doctors already boast of practicing "quality control" over "products of the womb" (i.e., babies) through genetic preselection. Gene-line "therapy" and cloning are not far behind (Davis-Floyd and Dumit, 1998). In addition to "designer babies" there are also, as we discussed earlier, designer drugs being developed by "cosmetic pharmacologists." These are nostrums marketed to those who are not certifiably diseased, but to normals, to make them feel "better than well."

Madness

If human beings are perennially discontented about their physical appearances this is even truer about their psychic states. From the beginning of history humans have used mind-altering intoxicants to transport themselves beyond the humdrum horizons of everydayness: fermented fruits, grains, and vegetables, selected leaves and needles, flowers of various sorts, roots, bulbs, and fungi. When chemical enhancement has not been surreptitiously promoted, governments and religions have railed against it.[3] And, as with campaigns against bodily mutilation, these recriminations have come to nothing. What is new, and for some commentators alarming, is a contemporary "furor psychopharmacologus" whose end, they fear, will be a society organized along the lines of Aldous Huxley's *Brave New World*, doped up on Soma (Chodoff, 2002, 628).

From its origins in the eighteenth century, psychiatry has had scientific pretensions. However, it wasn't until 1980, with the American Psychiatric Association's (APA's) publication of the third edition of its reference book, the *Diagnostic and Statistical Manual of Mental Disorders (DSM-III)*, that these dreams began to be realized in fact. Now for the first time psychic afflictions would be viewed, like physical diseases, as "internal pathologies that cause symptomatic behaviors" (Kutchins and Kirk, 1997, 40). The consequences of this have turned out to be monumental.

First, mental distresses were decontextualized. Their possible social and cultural etiologies were ignored and attention turned instead to consideration of "brain dysfunctions" and "chemical imbalances" that could be "managed."

Second, diagnostic criteria tested for reliability and validity were made available to psychiatrists, enabling them to differentiate one "syndrome" from another and therefore to prescribe precise treatment plans.

Third, as the ambiguous psychoanalytic concept of neurosis fell into disuse, there was an eruption of "mental diseases," each with their own slightly different symptomology (Spiegel, 2005, 61). Thus, while the second edition of the diagnostic manual (the *DSM-II*, issued in 1968) was only 134 pages long, the *DSM-III* (1980) contained nearly five hundred pages. The *DSM-IV*, published in 1994, boasts nine hundred pages and three hundred different "disease" classifications.

Fourth, what had for centuries been viewed as inescapable, if unpleasant, aspects of normal life became medically problematized (Chodoff, 2002, 662). If one was overly shy and introverted, they might now be diagnosed as a victim of social anxiety disorder (SAD). Or, if they experienced sweating and butterflies before a competition, a speech, or a job interview, then it was possible they had GAD, generalized anxiety disorder (for more examples, see table 4.1). For each of these there is list of recommended drugs, including for children.

A recent *New York Times* series reported a dramatic rise in medicinal "cocktails for kids," some as young as three, for temper tantrums, excitability, and fighting (Harris, 2006). A child might take Ritalin for concentration in the classroom; the anticonvulsive, Depokate, to control mood swings; the anti-psychotic, Risperdal, in the afternoon; and the hypnotic, Ambien, to put them to sleep at night. Parents are now being told that such regimens may have to be followed throughout the child's life. What the long-range consequences of this might be are still unknown; however, the preliminary signs are not encouraging (Silverman and Treisman, 2006).

One ironic aspect about these developments is that the *DSM-IV* purports to be "based on a phenomenological approach." This is because it presumably implements Edmund Husserl's admonition that investigators return "to things themselves," to factual descriptions of psychopathology with no theoretical or methodological presuppositions (Bracken and Thomas, 2005, 108–11). It should be obvious from what we have just said, however, that the *DSM-IV* bears little resemblance to our characterization of phenomenology. On the contrary, it merely extends the traditional scientific model, with all its prejudices, to the psyche.

To begin with, the *DSM-IV* lifts the patient out of his or her meaningful engagement with the world in order to provide a neutral diagnosis. It then offers a tableau of "methods" to be used in making these diagnoses. In this way it proceeds exactly as a scientist would: detaching a thing from its background so that it can be seen more clearly and objectively. Furthermore, and most importantly, it assumes that the self is a skin-encapsulated, biologically impelled "tinker-toy" collection of "data points" (Cushman, 2003, 108; Richardson et al., 1999). That is, instead of seeing human being as phenomenologists actually do, as a *way* of living in the world, as a unified field of daily cares and concerns (i.e., as *Leib*), it pictures it as *Körper*: an organism whose movements or "operants" are caused by electrical discharges and chemicals.

Physical Impairment

Anthropologists once defined human beings as toolmakers (*Homo fabricans*) to distinguish them from other beings. This demarcation is no longer plausible. Not only is toolmaking known to be widespread among chimpanzees, seagulls, and alligators; tools with "human" capabilities are now commonplace. Because of this, the question is once again being asked: What *is* the difference between "man and beast" *and* between "man and machine"?

Today there are mechanical devices with stereoscopic vision and the capacity to walk, swim, fly, snake along the ground, and sidle like crabs. Some can "talk" and others are able to "dance" or "play" with their human masters. Machines can be infected with "viruses" and can be engineered to repair and replicate, if not strictly reproduce, themselves, and they can be made to fabricate other, simpler, mechanical "species." The Gastrobot, as it is known, can even keep itself "alive" (i.e., moving) by incorporating "food," water, and air directly from the environment and eliminating its own waste. Other "bots" display the capacity to logically choose different courses of action based on the information they receive, and to do this more rapidly and with fewer errors than people. IBM's Deep Blue has defeated grandmaster Gary Kasparov at chess. There are now robot pets, robot couriers, and nursebots. There are robot therapists to treat autism and storybots that not only recite bedtime stories, but also act them out. And, of course, the reader is already familiar with robocops, robowarriors, and, soon to come, robocars that will be ridden, not driven (for photographs of these machines, see Aylett, 2002).

To be sure, the plastic and stainless steel coverings of these ingenious devices are hardly skins, but some bots are now being enshrouded in flexible, self-healing, touch-sensitive latex. True, pulleys and motors are poor equivalents to human muscles, but piezoelectric facsimiles made from electro-active polymers are now on the drawing board. Digital processors are as far from being neural networks as computers are from being brains. However, engineers promise that the differences between them will soon be bridged by means of artificial neural networks (ANNs): cultured neurons enclosed in computer chips. This will permit direct communication between brains and machines. Indeed, eel brains have already been linked to optical sensors and to robot wheel drives permitting the robots to "see" and move on command. Future war amputees can look forward to being outfitted with bionic limbs. The brains of military pilots will be directly hooked up to their planes' controls, permitting maneuverability solely through thought. The planes will essentially be extensions of their own bodies.

In short, according to Donna Haraway, the age of the cyborg has commenced! (1991, 149–81). La Mettrie's centuries-old proposition has proven true: man is a machine after all. Haraway writes of "transgressed boundaries, potent fusions, and dangerous possibilities" (154), of mechanical humanoids, of mind-body fusion, and of the integration of male and female body parts: "In a sense, organisms have ceased to exist as objects of knowledge, giving way to biotic components, i.e., special kinds of information-processing devices" (164). One of these is the moody robot known as Kismet.

According to bioengineers an emotion is in essence a series of bodily gestures. And the basic movements associated with joy, sadness, fear, and the like have now been entered into a so-called facial coding system (FACS). "Happy," for example, is signified by a smile. A smile in turn requires two specific "action units" (AUs): a "lip corner puller" and a "cheek raiser." Or, to express it in FACS terms, "Happy$_{df}$ = AU12 + AU6" (Aylett, 2002, 108). Once these movements are programmed into a computer that has been affixed with a latex-skin face and piezoelectric muscles, it will be capable of consorting intelligently with us. Or, if that seems like too much, take the more prosaic case of a soldier whose face has been mangled in battle. He or she can now be re-equipped with a prosthetic face fully capable of emoting. If, in addition, this face is implanted with ANNs, the emotions will be subject to the wounded veteran's directions. Other impairments such as quadriplegia and blindness will be treated in comparable ways.

Getting Real

If there is something menacing in the idea that we are destined to being wedded to machines, it is an unease shared by William Gibson in *Neuromancer*, wherein cumbersome human "meat" is surgically displaced by the crystalline purity of computers. But because they are already so deeply implicated in our lives, from our pacemakers, digital day planners, cell phones, and cars to our sanitary water supplies, foodstuffs, and electrical grids, it is difficult to articulate our concern. This is where phenomenology can help. To show how, we can turn to the preeminent trans-humanist fantasy, one that makes nano-medicine, organ transplants, and cyber-tots "look like hiccoughs" (Mander, 1991, 183): the quest for immortality.

Let us assume that self-consciousness is reducible to data stored in the brain, says Hans Moravec, director of the Mobile Robot Laboratory at Carnegie Mellon University. This being the case, then it should be capable of being digitally downloaded onto a hard disk of a supercomputer (Moravec, 1988). When this is accomplished then our organic bodies, destined for death, could be discarded like last year's passé clothing fashion. The "I" would be re-housed in a shiny new machine with an eternal warranty. Patients, we are assured, will have their choice of console color. As to objections that human brains calculate at rates one thousand times faster than any known computer, this is dismissed by Moravec as a mere technical difficulty. From 1910 to 1990 alone there was a trillionfold decline in the cost of mechanical calculation. And estimates are that as their sizes fall in the next fifty years, the speed of computers will dramatically accelerate. A more pressing question concerns whether the "I" really is a "data pattern" that can be represented by a series of binary notations: 1 and 0. In other words, can the "I" be beamed down by a *Star Trek*–like Scotty? Wouldn't something be lost in the transmission? Once again, the news is comforting: "You (i.e., 'I') are only your mind, or 'your pattern,' which . . . can be transmitted into a machine . . . or two or three or many machines. . . . That is, the real you can be infinitely duplicated," as can those of any other animate life form. And all without "the awful limits of flesh" (Moravec, paraphrased in Mander, 1991, 186).

Moravec predicts that very soon, a "robot brain surgeon," bristling with "microscopic machinery and a cable" will be able to expose your brain, "place a hand on its surface" and then, layer by layer, extricate the thing called "you" (i.e., "I"). But phenomenologically speaking, this makes little sense because the "I" is not an object that occupies a specific geographic location inside the body. It is, as we have repeatedly pointed out, a *how*. It is *the way* we experience ourselves for the most part in the world, the way we are "there" (*Da*) in lived time and space. And the testimony of our lived experience, unmediated by theories of physical chemistry or bedazzled by electronic wizardry, teaches us the following: I may indeed be a binary "pattern" in my brain, as Moravec claims; however, "I" am also in my heart (as a poet might say). And "I" am housed in the lower depths of my belly, the *dan tien* point, as the Japanese Buddhist would insist, where it is on display for public viewing by means of a gruesome operation known as *seppuku* (i.e., *hara kiri* = belly slitting). Or, more prosaically, "I" am in my leg and toe. In other words, the "I" infuses my entire flesh. It is *con*-fused with my body, *is* my body. *I am my body.* Only during those rare moments when its smooth functioning falters and I can no longer trust the body's parts to work do they become visible to me as objects separate from "me": when the brain no longer remembers names, when the heart shudders to a stop, when the leg no longer bears weight, or the aching toe keeps me awake. Otherwise, "so long as we feel well, ['I'] do not exist. More exactly: we do not know that we exist" (Cioran, in Morris, 2000, 50).

As a *way* of being-in-the-world, I am not contained inside a skin capsule. On the contrary, the "I" extends far beyond its fleshly housing into the world of space and time. To be sure, there are moments during which I become conscious of a separation or isolation from my surroundings. But this occurs when the current of our shared life is disrupted by an untoward act, by your objectifying gaze, by a novel situation (say, a job interview or a first date), or by a crisis of some sort. Only then, when the predictability of our togetherness vanishes, do I become visible to myself *as* a unique self. Up to that time we are, as Merleau-Ponty would say, "common flesh." Not billiard balls bumping against each other, but *persons* mutually "undergoing" each others' odors, physicality, touch, and voicing. In this state we are immediately (i.e., without the mediation of our minds) turned on, repelled, put at ease, or on guard.

The logical end of enhancement medicine is to treat death as a disease: to extend the length of time allotted to us, eternally. And like all previous quests along these lines, it takes time for granted as a natural fact with an existence independent of us. Phenomenology radically shifts the problematic of time. In doing so, it calls into question this project. It undermines it by asking not *what* time is, but *who* time is (Heidegger, 1992, 4).

According to Heidegger, there is an *in*authentic time experience. Here, time is thought and seen as a "what": a linear continuum. Then there is "primordial" or authentic temporality: *my* time, when I realize that *I* am time. Inauthentic time is sensed as a succession of now-points flying by like cars speeding down the interstate, disappearing into the past. It is something we can "run out of" and, with the aid of technology, "extend." *My* time is different. It is the "movement" (*Bewegung*) of my own life as it unfolds, ceaselessly pressing forward into future possibilities, bringing in its wake memories of the past. Here, the future is not an indeterminate "not yet present" on an imaginary timeline. It is the open horizon of anticipated goals and undertakings. When I am young and vigorous, my future is rich and wide; it holds any number of choices and opportunities. There will be the trip to Europe, the job I always wanted, a fulfilling relationship. As I age this horizon gradually shrinks. Adventures once eagerly planned for shade into fantasies. Finally, they darken into impossibilities. Puberty, fertility, pregnancy, menopause, decrepitude are inevitable phases in *my* time, moments in *my* life. This being so, it is more than just a minor philosophical error to associate them with the "bad" or the "ill" that comprise part of the Greek meaning of *dys*, as in "disorder" (Svaneaus, 2000, 98). It is a betrayal of my time, my being.

The point, then, is not that biomechanical engineers cannot build human-like robots capable of "emoting," that pharmaceutical companies cannot mix magical elixirs, or that we are incapable of designing nanosecond computers whose calculating power rivals that of the human brain. The question is, rather, *my* end? Surely, none of these technological innovations can put an end to our finitude. Maybe they can mitigate our immediate pains, but they never relieve us of existential suffering. For just below the comfortable surface of my workday routines lies an inner quaking—the painful awareness that I am moving toward not-being, that I am coming to an end. The more insistently this realization breaks into my consciousness, the more frantic are my efforts at suppression. It is precisely those most serene in their self-assuredness, most affably glib, most certain that life can be painlessly extended indefinitely, who are most in denial about their own death, and who are therefore most guilty of betrayal (Becker, 1973, 178–80; Becker, 1975, 158).

Notes

1. In an attempt to surpass the received notion of immaterial mind separated from material body (and the philosophical difficulties implied by it), Edmund Husserl argued that there is no such event as consciousness in the abstract. Rather, consciousness is always "intentional." It is always directed toward one object or another. Thus, perception is always, "of something, recalling of something, thinking of something, hoping for something, fearing something . . . and so on" (Husserl, 1996, 15). Likewise, Heidegger's notion of care: it is never without that to which it is directed.

2. In contrast, at least in *Being and Time*, Heidegger's observations are borrowed largely from Søren Kierkegaard and his ruminations about nineteenth-century bourgeois life in Copenhagen.

3. Cf. the failed war against tobacco undertaken by the Ottoman Empire, see Szasz (1975, 173).

8

Recovering Therapy

In his 1946 essay, "Letter on Humanism," Heidegger writes these cryptic lines: "Language is the house of being. In its home man dwells" (1977b, 193). Here, Heidegger is not using "language" in the conventional sense, as a medium to convey information about objects, or as a system of word-sounds that refer to specific feelings, thoughts, or things. Indeed, for Heidegger language is not necessarily *linguistic* at all (Guignon, 1983, 111–12). Rather, language is taken to mean a shared context of meaning (or, as anthropologists might say, a "deep culture") that enables things—humans, trees, cars, jobs, relationships, and the like—to show up as they do, in intelligible ways: for a woman to appear *as* a friend, for example, a tree *as* shade, a BMW *as* a status symbol, a job *as* a means of security, and so on. It is this background of shared meanings that allows us to understand verbal utterances, writings, and physical gestures; that enables us to use the same upturned lips to communicate affection to one person, while conveying contempt for another; to use the same words to send one message to a student and an entirely different one to our spouse. In short, it is only on the basis of "dwelling" in a particular language that things make sense to us; they become what they are.

Due to the prestige of the natural sciences, the prevailing context of meaning today is technological. As a result, our relationships to things, including people, tend to be instrumental.

They show up as "standing reserves" (*Bestanden*) of objects awaiting manipulation and transformation by the human subject. Although the modern term "technology" can be traced back to the ancient Greek word *technē*, according to Heidegger it has lost much of its original resonance. *Technē*, he says, captures the idea of "revealing" things or "bringing [things] forth," as a sculptor or a farmer might, who help "release" what is already potentially in the stone or the seed, making it possible for them to become, respectively, a statue or a crop. To illustrate, Heidegger cites the case of the premodern craftsman who builds "the old wooden bridge" that "*lets* the river run its course" (Heidegger, 1977a, 16; Heidegger, 1977d, 330, our emphasis). This is in contrast to the instrumentalist technology of a hydroelectric dam that *forces* the river into a reservoir so that it can be utilized as "water power." As Heidegger sees it, modern technology compels things to be revealed in only one way, as resources to be rationally "set upon," "challenged," and "enframed" (*Gestell*).

Technological language has had a decisive and highly problematic impact on the healing professions. For ancient Greek physicians, healing was understood as *technē*, the artful practice of aiding the body in restoring itself back to its natural condition of harmony. By the twentieth century healing was well on the way to becoming a "military machine" (*machine á guerir*), to quote Michel Foucault (Greco, 1998, 66), wherein the body is viewed, not as a self-healing whole, but as an object, a hindrance to be mastered and made-over after design specifications. Thus, while for Socrates, physicians were admonished to be like skilled rhetoricians, adapting their treatments to what is called for given what they know of the patient's biography (*Phaedrus*, 270b, c), the job of the modern doctor has increasingly become one of fitting patients into preset standards of corporeal functioning, occasionally *regardless* of the patient's personal needs and requirements.[1] Instead of a person who suffers, in other words, they are viewed as a "a litany of [objective] facts—surgery dates, complications endured, disease statistics, etc." (Ogle, 2001). As a case in point, consider the following observations.

In referring to an infant's death at a conference on child mortality, Renée Anspach reports one discussant describing their patient this way: "Baby girl Simpson was the 10,344-gram product of a 27-week gestation." The mother is "a 21-year-old Gravida III, Para I, AbI black female." Here, the baby is no longer the child of a grieving mother but the "product" of a womb. The mother in turn is reduced to a series of impersonal numbers and codes that depict her age, previous pregnancies, live births, abortions, race, and weeks of pregnancy (Anspach, 1994, 319).[2]

Anspach goes on to describe how objectification is amplified by use of the passive voice typical of medical experts. Passive voicing rhetorically eliminates the presence of an active agent who actually makes diagnostic and therapeutic decisions. Thus, the doctor reports that "the infant was transferred. . . ," "She was treated with high FiO2's [respirator settings]. . . ," "She was extubated" (taken off the respirator), "was transferred here," or "was put on phenobarb" (320). In these statements, *what* was done is emphasized, rather than *who* did it. With no human decision maker to point to, the issues of accountability waft away like smoke. Instead, responsibility falls on the technology. The instrumentality of the laboratory becomes the "active agent": the computed axial tomography (the CAT scan), for example, not the doctor who uses it (321). The authority of technology in medical decision making is mirrored in subtle linguistic inflections like these: "follow-up CAT-scans have *shown* the amount of blood flow to be minimal," "The arteriogram *reveals* that this AVM was fed," "The EEG *showed* . . . an abnormal," and so on (321).

Just as the doctor as an agent disappears from medical decision making as the authority of his or her equipment increases, the patient also becomes invisible. The personal account of his or her condition comes to be regarded as a subjective, thus presumably biased, narrative of "symptoms." Thus, the patient is said to "report" that she has been taking her medication, to "state" that she does not smoke or drink. Because their bias is assumed, such statements and reports are routinely dismissed in favor of objective *signs*. Medical signs are considered "hard facts." These are restricted to what can be "noted," "observed," or "found" by means of standardized laboratory tests (Anspach 1994, 324; Kleinman, 1988, 214; Jewson, 1976).

Two generations ago the severity of coronary heart disease (CHD), or "hardening of the arteries," was assessed by inquiring into the patient's ability to walk up stairs and to work. For adult males (but not necessarily women), the existence of a heart attack proper (a cardiac infarction) was confirmed by reports of crushing pain issuing down one's left arm, cold sweat, and nausea. Today, such accounts are considered preliminary, at best, to objective laboratory tests. The progression of CHD is assessed through catheterization of the femoral artery and an angiography that produces X-rays of the heart. An infarction is verified by the presence of cardiac enzymes in the bloodstream and/or by jagged alpha waves on an electrocardiogram readout; or, more recently, by echocardiography and radionuclide cineangiography (Feinstein, 1983).

Today, many doctors struggle with the dilemma into which medical technology has thrust them. They readily grant that it enhances their capacity to deal with the *Körper*, the human organism and its pathologies. But they resent how it interferes with their desire to care for living persons with their own moods, choices, and relationships.[3] Here is the confession of one physician:

> I work hard at keeping up with the latest developments. I want to be technically first rate. After all, that's what patients need. But that is only the mechanical aspect of care. I feel what really counts is the human aspect. That is both a lot tougher and lot more rewarding. . . . Entering patients' life worlds and listening to their pain, helping them make sense of their suffering, helping them to cope with the burden of disease—all that is what makes my work rewarding. (Kleinman, 1988, 213)

A colleague concurs with this, and offers the following rather dismal forecast of his profession's future: "I don't know what will happen to the [personal] side of medicine as we make medical practice so highly technical and so dominated by cost accounting, bureaucratic rules, and an adversarial relationship with patients. . . . In my darker moments I think we are at the end of medicine as we know it" (Kleinman, 1988, 215–16; Freund et al., 2003, 247–49).[4]

Toward Phenomenology

As pointed out in the first chapter, one of the goals of phenomenology is to "de(con)struct" or dismantle traditional scientific
presuppositions concerning human being and the medical authority based on them. But phenomenology can also be *con-
structive* by re-envisioning the healing arts. There are a number
of encouraging signs of just such a turn. Take the psychoneu-
roimmunology of George Engel, for example (Engel, 1977; 1980).

Engel emphasizes how disease symptoms reflect not only
the body's physiological mechanics, but also how the person in-
terprets their internal states. This, in turn, is partly a product of
their biography as well as their cultural inheritance (O'Connor,
2005, 59–60). Like us, for instance, Chinese people suffer fatigue,
poor appetite, and insomnia. They lose interest in life and complain of boredom. However, to admit to having a Western condition like depression would open them to stigmatizing
sanctions. In any case, Chinese physicians are not trained to recognize these body signals as symptoms of depression, and there
is no word in Chinese medical jargon strictly translatable to it
(O'Connor, 2005, 60). What this suggests, according to Engel, is
that the same bodily indicators may point to one condition in
Asian culture, while having an entirely different meaning to us.

The therapeutic implications of this observation can be seen
in the orientation of Viktor von Weisäcker. Although he was
trained as a physiologist, Weisäcker repudiated conventional
theories of psychosomatic medicine, specifically the notion that
one's psychic state can aggravate or actually cause a disease.
This style of psychosomatics, he believed, merely extends the
naturalistic explanation of disease to include one more causal element—the psyche—and a minor one at that. As to its practical
ameliorative effects, Weisäcker concluded that essentially they
add up to "nothing at all" (Greco, 1998, 78).[5]

Weisäcker was skeptical of biologically reductive disease
models because he believed that human being in the phenomenological sense cannot be considered a composite of material
substances. Nor can a human ailment ever be taken simply as an
objective event that befalls an organism. Thus, the proper role of

a phenomenologically informed psychosomatics must involve more than eliminating organic pathologies. It should also assist patients in negotiating the various life crises in which they find themselves. Today, German internists treating patients who present with otherwise inexplicable symptoms—say, severe digestive problems or chronic pain—can be certified to administer psychosomatic protocols in order to determine whether, for example, they have been traumatized. Comparable developments can also be witnessed in continental European psychology and psychiatry.

Disenchanted with the mechanistic viewpoint that had come to dominate their professions in England and America by the early 1940s, a group of prominent German and Swiss practitioners—including Medard Boss, Roland Kuhn, and Ludwig Binswanger—devised an alternative therapy called *Daseinsanalyse*, after the Heideggerian interpretation of human existence as *Dasein*. Just as Weisäcker had insisted that a bona fide "anthropological" psychosomatics would address how patients are in-the-world, practitioners of Daseinsanalyse believe that mental troubles should be dealt with in the same way, as expressions of socially constructed character defenses that serve to protect individuals from the impermanence and fragility of existence. Daseinsanalyse does not inquire into the causes of a patient's "pathologic idiosyncrasies according to the teachings of . . . psychotherapy, or by means of its preferred categories." Rather, it attempts to understand these idiosyncrasies as "modifications of the total structure" of their culturally and historically situated existence (Binswanger, 1956, 145; May, 1967).

The groundbreaking work of biomedical scientist Jon Kabat-Zinn (1990), mentioned in the first chapter, provides still another example of an attempt to ground medical care phenomenologically. He calls his program mindfulness-based stress reduction (MBSR). By regarding the patient as a whole person rather than as a collection of quantifiable data points, MBSR does not focus principally on *what* is wrong with the machine-body, but with *how* the patient is living in an age of technologically accelerated sensory arousal. At the heart of MBSR are "mindfulness practices," based on Buddhist meditation models. These include pay-

ing attention to one's own stress-inducing behaviors and thinking habits, and "listening" to their internal body signals. According to Kabat-Zinn, these practices are clinically effective in
reducing some of the more debilitating symptoms of chronic illness discussed in chapter 6, especially pain.[6] Even if this is doubtful, they have the additional benefit of empowering patients with
skills to help them cope with self-defeating ways of being-in-the-
world. This, he believes, is superior to regarding them as passive
objects available for pharmacological quick fixes.

Hermeneutic Dialogue

Phenomenologically based psychotherapy urges patients to
come to grips with the precariousness of their condition. Instead
of prescribing pills to suppress their intuitive suspicion that
lurking just beneath the stability of their everyday lives is an
abyss of historical contingency and existential uncertainty, phenomenology calls patients to awaken to this fact. One of the
ways it does this is through what Hans-Georg Gadamer calls
hermeneutic dialogue (HD) (cf. Richardson et al., 1999, 60–76).
HD is best understood not as a therapy entire to itself, but as a
helpful adjunct to treatment strategies already being used by at
least some therapists.

Let us say that a client comes to the office complaining of
malaise and emptiness. The therapist using HD may begin by inquiring into recent traumas. Have they divorced, lost their job,
filed for bankruptcy? The point here is not to help the therapist
devise a treatment plan to "get the client going again." It is, instead, to compel the client to begin questioning their life choices
and commitments. For it is the various roles and identities they
cling to that create a false sense of stability, security, and permanence. As a case in point, when I proclaim "I am a professor," "a
happily married mother," "a competent worker with a sizable
nest egg," and so forth, I fool myself into thinking that I am solid
and grounded, that I am "realized," real. The therapist's job is to
gently, if insistently, disabuse me of this illusion. It is to *disillu-
sion* me, to get me to see that life is fundamentally, irrevocably,

fragile and precarious. Much like the Hindu meditative practice of *Neti, Neti*—"not this, not this"—which systematically destabilizes conviction in various illusions I may have about my own substantiality, HD awakens clients to the void at their very core: I am not my job, nor my awards, my lithe body, my thoughts, my bank account and properties. Rather, I am naught; I am no particular thing at all. In annihilating one's self-sureties, the client is opened to a new, heightened appreciation of life in all its mystery and preciousness.

Like an ethnographer, the therapist follows the thread laid down by clients, allowing them to reveal what matters to them in their (the clients') terms. Well-trained ethnographers consult the myths, art, dance, dress, and music of their subjects in order to grasp their community life. Just so, the skilled practitioner of HD might access their clients' diary confessions, poetry, and accounts of their workday lives (Campo, 2003). This, among other reasons, to uncover various "defense mechanisms," as they are called by psychoanalysts, people use to protect their bruised egos: overcompensation, scapegoating, "reaction formation" (hating what one cannot have), somatizing, sarcasm, and so on.

At first these tactics may not be entirely clear either to the client or the therapist. But by way of the latter's "What is this?" "Why do you say that?" "What does it mean to you?" "How do you feel about it?" their significance becomes clearer. Eventually, again like the ethnographer, the therapist comes to "stand 'there'" in the client's shoes, so to say; begins to see the world from the client's standpoint. In the tradition of hermeneutic phenomenology, the word for this kind of understanding is *Verstehen*. Wilhelm Dilthey describes *Verstehen* as "the rediscovery of the 'I' in the 'thou'" (Dilthey, 1961, 39).

HD does not offer a causal explanation of a patient's "mental disease" à la biomedicine. Nor does it seek to attain sympathy, a state of emotional mergence with the client: weeping as they weep, raging as they do, delighting in their pleasure, and the like. Instead, it is something closer to empathy. That is, the therapists imaginatively project what they know of their own mental contents onto the client. Their sincere "I see now," "I understand," "okay," presumably helps lead the client to self-understanding (*Sichverstehen*) (Gadamer, 1994, 254–64).

Dilthey, on whose teachings HD is partly based, believed that hermeneutic investigations could reach the foundational bedrock of a person's lived experience. HD, however, makes no such claims. It is understood at the outset that any interpretation of another's mental state is always colored by a "fore-structure" of assumptions that a therapist already brings to the situation; therefore any such interpretation is partial, provisional, and open-ended. There are multiple ways to make sense of another's anguish, and different questions by different therapists will bring out previously "undetermined possibilities" of meaning (Gadamer, 1994, 268). And yet, while therapists can never entirely eliminate their own biases and prejudices, they can nonetheless attempt to "own" them. In other words, they can be conscious of them so that the client's story "can present itself in all its otherness and assert its own truth against [them]" (269).

During the course of HD, the goal is for both therapist and client to "lose" themselves in the communicative "to and fro," as they move toward understanding. By remaining flexible and sensitive to the true otherness of the client's experience, the therapist is prepared to suspend professionally ingrained assumptions about the occasions of human suffering. But to do this well, a premium is placed on two qualities.

First is active listening—the cultivation of a capacity actually "to *hear* what the other is saying" (Gadamer, 1994, 316). The art of "giving ear" to the other is exactly what is too easily stifled by the diagnostic protocols recommended by the *DSM*, wherein "instead of learning to look for illness in the eyes of the patient or to listen for it in the patient's voice, [the doctor] tries to read off the data provided by technologically sophisticated measuring instruments" (Gadamer, 1996, 98). In HD the truth of mental illness is not to be found in objective measurement, but in what Gadamer describes as the "in-between," where two "horizons of understanding"—those of therapist and patient—are woven together, and where both of them are transformed as a result (Gadamer, 1996, 109).

The second quality is experience. Georg Simmel once said it this way: while one need never have been Caesar to understand Caesar, it is equally true that "whoever has never loved will never understand love or the lover; someone with a passionate disposition will never understand one who is apathetic. The weakling will never understand the hero, nor will the hero understand the weakling" (Simmel, 1977, 65). In other words, the more provincial and limited the therapist's own background and horizons are, the more difficult it will be for him to truly enter the lifeworld of the patient. To rephrase a popular cliché: good intentions notwithstanding, if one has not "walked the walk," they will find it virtually impossible to "understand the talk." The celibate will be hard pressed to counsel a person with sexual problems, the abstemious to understand the agonies of addiction. Psychotherapist Richard O'Connor suggests that therapists who have never gone through a serious depressive episode have no business treating depression. Likewise, if one has never faced his own existential emptiness, he can hardly be expected to aid the patient to grasp their own (O'Connor, 2005).

Notes

1. Socrates argues that "the method of the science of medicine is, I suppose, the same as that of the science of rhetoric." For just as it would be nonsense to say that persuasive speech is simply a matter of the "knack and experience" of using tropes and similes, it would be "madness" to say that a doctor is merely one who "knows how to apply things to bodies" to make them warm or cool, to make them vomit, or their bowels to move. These are no more than the "preliminaries" of health care, not its essential "element."

2. For a further illuminating example, see Freund et al. (2003, 243–48).

3. Eric Cassell (1991) provides a brilliant portrayal of the dilemma facing medicine,

4. The crisis is not merely a historical byproduct of a technological worldview. It also grows out of specific market forces in the West that have helped to change the landscape of health care delivery. With the appearance of managed care organizations (MCOs), regulatory bureaucratic processes and objectifying economic strategies have become mandatory for the financial survival of physicians if they want reimbursement from insurance companies. For more on this, see chapter 3.

5. For more on the differences between empirically inclined, scientistic Anglo-American psychiatry and its German counterpart, see the illuminating discussion by Monica Greco (1998, esp. 73–92).

6. In September 2004, Kabat-Zinn's program celebrated its twenty-fifth year in continual operation, with over sixteen thousand medical patients having completed the eight-week program. Kabat-Zinn claims that MBSR can help change the neural pathways in the brain that spawn conditions like anxiety and depression.

9

Conclusion

Today, American medicine finds itself in a highly competitive market as large numbers of dissatisfied patients are talking with their feet and migrating en masse to alternative health care providers. Already, as early as 1993 *The New England Journal of Medicine* was reporting that allopathic physicians (M.D.s) were losing $13.7 billion annually to chiropractors, acupuncturists, and naturopaths. Most of this was coming from the patients' own pocketbooks (Eisenberg et al., 1993). The result is that medicine has been compelled to be more self-critical (Anderson, 2001).

In one forum medical doctors urge each other to "lurk" online, "listen to," and "learn from" discussions about consumer demands (Chin, 2003). In another, doctors air doubts about what passes as medical knowledge, confessing that there are "a few things we know, a few we think we know (but probably don't), and lots of things we don't know" (McAlister, 2003). In still other places, they share stories about "patients like Linda," who suffer from medically undiagnosed diseases (MUDs) such as benign chronic intractable pain (Ringel, 2003). They warn each other to take more care with their word choices and to exhibit behaviors reminiscent of what we described in the last chapter as hermeneutic dialogue (Bedell et al., 2004).

To be sure, there remains a residue of grumbling among physicians about "spoiled patients" (Hughes, 2003), "noncompliant patients," and the necessity to "manage challenging encounters" so that patients will "make the 'best' choices" (read: those consistent with biomedical interests) (Martinez, 2003; McNutt, 2004). In reaction to defiant patients, we come across surprisingly defensive outbursts by those "who did, after all, go to medical school" (Anderson, 2001). Yet just beneath the surface of the doctors' in-house discussions lies an ironic subtext: a kind of medical cultism flourishing not just among professionals, but also within the lay community. In other words, at the very moment when thoughtful physicians are beginning to question the epistemic foundations of their own explanatory models, many lay people are embracing the ontology of the *Körper* with more fervor than ever. The public at large is increasingly coming to share a conviction that their own bodily troubles are entirely explicable (and treatable) in biomechanical terms.

One of the most notable indicators of lay medical cultism is the growing insistence by patients, often in the face of resistance by doctors, that their bodily complaints be framed with a medical label (Fischoff and Wesseley, 2003; Barker, 2002; Brown et al., 2000; Kroll-Smith and Floyd, 1997). Often the patients in question are articulate middle-class married females between the ages of forty and sixty years, with biographies of anxiety, and habits of self-catastrophizing. Plagued with chronic diarrhea, joint pains, exhaustion, and hives, "driven by fear of the unknown, [they] are happy to finally receive a [medical] diagnosis that could account for their symptoms" (Hassett and Sigal, 2002, 1812). Far from being reassured by negative laboratory findings that show no biological basis for their complaints, they demand further testing. Doctors who accede to their wishes do so reluctantly given that more tests can "expose patients to iatrogenic [physician-induced] harm and amplify symptoms" (Barsky and Borus, 1999). However, from a practical financial standpoint they are reluctant *not* to do so because these same patients are also typically the best insured. To this we can add the justified terror American physicians have of litigious lawyers.

Doctors who dig in their heels and say no to patients, or who dare dismiss their complaints with replies like "it's all in your head" or "you're being hysterical" can anticipate far more than simply being ignored. When Elaine Showalter wrote *Hystories* (1997), in which she sociologically deconstructed what she referred to as "hysterical epidemics" like chronic fatigue syndrome, Gulf War syndrome, and multiple personality disorder, she was besieged with hate mail, one writer threatening to "rip her apart" (x).

Two conclusions can be drawn from these observations. One is that when it comes to explaining and treating body troubles, infinitely more is at stake than neutral academic considerations. Second, contrary to what medical critic Ivan Illich suggests in *Medical Nemesis* (1976), it is profoundly inaccurate and unfair to attribute the movement to medicalize the human condition to a conspiracy of "bio-fascists." On the contrary, it is increasingly evident that all of us in one way or another are complicit in reproducing medicalization through our own, semi-conscious, daily practices.

The most probable culprit behind heightened lay expectations of what medicine can do is the ubiquitous hospital TV series that depicts sixty-minute miracle cures of deadly afflictions by teams of square-jawed actors and their buxom attendants. Added to this is the ease of self-diagnostics provided by Internet websites and by the untold thousands of support groups, blogs, and chat rooms available online to sufferers. Gesine Küspert estimates that there are 182,000 such sources for victims of chronic fatigue, 126,000 for fibromyalgiacs, 84,200 for those plagued with irritable bowels, and a mind-boggling 343,000 for those with multiple chemical sensitivity (Küspert, 2006, 33). And these concern only MUDs! The number of online resources available to those with bona fide diseases is many times greater than this (totaling 1.3+ million for AIDS sufferers alone) (34). Nor can we overlook mentioning the explosion in direct-to-consumer drug and surgery advertisements, with their shorthand lists of symptoms and tiny enumerations of (sometimes lethal) side effects. Finally, there is the abundant insurance compensation available to those who can have their afflictions certified with what one cynical internist has called a "delightful me too disorder," for example, whiplash (cf. Malleson, 2002).[1]

As compelling as these explanations for medical cultism are there is another, more fundamental, consideration, one that we have already alluded to several times in earlier chapters. It is the existential fact of our own finitude, and the ways by which our bodies somatize it through muscle aches, runny bowels, choking sensations, heart palpitations, boredom, and panic. These body signs, coupled with a growing disbelief in conventional religious means of redemption, have given rise to fantasies of medical salvation. Just as belief in alien abduction, satanic ritual abuse, or cosmic terrorism vividly articulate an ultimately inarticulable truth, so does the fetishism of disease. By this, we mean the conviction that my impermanence, my emptiness, is caused by a biomechanical dysfunction that can be fixed by going to the doctor. Flying saucers, Bigfoot, black magic, and medicine function today as culturally acceptable, occasionally destructive "iconic social communications" for those "not . . . able to speak or even to admit what they feel" (Showalter, 1997, 7). They are shorthand codes that, with varying degrees of sophistication and empirical support, express the abyss at our very core.

Ordinarily the endless circus of work and shopping serve their intended purpose. They relieve us of having to be alone with our own fragility and vulnerability, allowing us to "take our ease," as Martin Heidegger might say. However, when they fail to secure the scaffolding erected above the swirling darkness, we feel something is not quite right. At that point nonspecific angst turns into fear of a particular thing: of stranger danger, perhaps, of extraterrestrials, of weapons of mass destruction, or Internet predators. In our era, increasingly it transmogrifies into the feeling that something is wrong with *me*, that I'm not well. I'm sick and need to see a doctor.

We challenge readers to face the truth that while biomedicine can and has accomplished wondrous things, there is one thing it can never do. It can never put an end to the precariousness endemic to life: a condition of which all of us, in quiet moments, are intuitively aware. Ignoring the instances when they have actual biological sources, our gastric distress, our tiredness, muscle pains, anxieties, despair, and rage are inevitable dimensions of human being. They can no more be fixed than death can.

We also encourage health care professionals to continue questioning the assumption that their diagnostic categories and technologies are unambiguously objective and neutral. To say it simply, objectivity is impossible when it comes to the situated complexity of human being. Far from being neutral and trans-historical, the diagnostic instrumentality of modern medicine is *itself* historically constructed and culturally relative. In short, the movement of history determines in advance what is worthy of our attention.

Finally, we urge proponents of managed care organizations (MCOs) who seem convinced that speed, technical efficiency, and cost-effectiveness result in more equitable and better quality health care to come clean. MCO regulations almost always look past the "text," as we call it, that gives meaning to people's lives and that, occasionally, deforms their bodies.

To repeat, we are not saying that there are no curable body troubles, or that either technological biomedicine or the MCO industry are irrelevant or without value. While their benefits are often exaggerated (Markle and McCrea, 2008), it is unassailable that modern diagnostics, new medications, and surgeries can save and sometimes enhance life.

Take the case of suicidal depression. The first stage of an elaborate series of drug trials known as STAR*D, conducted earlier in this century, found that serotonin reuptake inhibitors like Celexa actually have few depression-relieving effects. However, during the second stage, when Celexa was augmented with an additional anti-depressant such as Buspar or Wellbutrin, there was a measurable increase in remission rates (Trivedi et al., 2006). The reader should bear in mind that because no placebo controls were used in the STAR*D study, it remains an open question as to whether the drugs are more effective than sugar pills (although independent data show that they are [cf. Reynolds (2006)]).[2] More importantly, we should remember that the STAR*D experiments do not answer whether a two-drug combination is more successful in treating depression than cognitive therapy (CT) might be, and/or behavioral activation therapy (BA).[3] (Findings from a number of experiments suggest that CT and BA are at least as effective in this regard as pharmaceuticals [Dimidjian et al., 2006; DeRubeis et al., 1999].) But even granted that a two- (or, as some researchers are now proposing, a three-) drug cocktail can reduce major depression, the practice of relying on medicine is in itself, to us, a disturbing trend. For it habituates us to comprehend ourselves and our ailments in bio-mechanical terms. True, we are endowed with corporeal flesh, an organism that occasionally becomes pathological. But the method of phenomenology tells us that the *how* of lived pain and suffering do not emerge from corporeal dysfunctions alone. Nor can they be adequately treated as if they do. Rather, physical and psychological agonies are constituted partly by how we are meaningfully engaged in the world. And this is because we are infinitely more than isolated physical objects. Instead, we are "inextricably woven together," as Merleau-Ponty would say, into a larger cultural-historical unity. Furthermore, we are unique in being at least tacitly aware of our finitude, and we always make sense of this realization in terms of our relations with others who share this same discomfiting knowledge. Thus, we should never be treated simply as "cases" to be measured, causally explained, and controlled. The practice of hermeneutic dialogue, described in the last chapter, takes place between *persons* who are deeply attentive to each other, persons who place demands on each other, and who respond to each other as ends in themselves, not just as paying customers or as vendors of marketable commodities.

In order for medicine to be recovered as a truly humane science, it will be necessary for all of us to acknowledge that the cultural-historical complexity of the human condition can never be collapsed into a universal "nature"; one amenable to a single "method" which, if followed correctly, will result in some sort of "objective" truth. But again, our argument is not that science is the "problem." The problem, as Heidegger says, is uncritically applying the fixed rules of the natural sciences to everything, including the situated finitude of human existence (2001a, 134). The strict emphasis on method that modern medicine typically abides by continues to cut us off from a deeper sense of truth. This is the truth of our own lived experience, which, as Gadamer reminds us, "transcends the sphere of the scientific method" (Gadamer, 1994, xxii). The experience of being cut off in this way has the pernicious effect of frustrating, angering, and fostering distrust in both patient and doctor toward each other—which is ironic given that patients yearn for help from doctors, and doctors equally want to provide it. Thus, while pharmaceuticals and elaborate diagnostic technologies must never be ruled out, the first priority of a truly humane science of health care must always be to attend to the lived patient and his/her way of being-in-the-world.

Notes

1. For the ongoing debate in medical journals concerning the role played by insurance companies in the reification of medical labels, see Küspert (2006, 261–62).

2. For more on STAR*D, see chapter 2, note 3.

3. Cognitive therapy deals with depression by encouraging patients to become aware of and rid themselves of self-defeating thought patterns. Behavioral therapy ignores the content of thoughts and focuses instead on self-destructive behaviors like overscheduling, the avoidance of uncomfortable situations, and so on.

Appendix

The Phenomenon of Phenomenology

In 1882, German philosopher Friedrich Nietzsche published the first edition of *The Gay Science,* a book of aphorisms that struck Germany and much of Europe like a bolt of lightning, undermining the deepest values and convictions of Western thought. One aphorism concerns a madman who, after years of serene isolation in the mountains, descends into the city. He enters the bustling market in the early morning and, amid the throng of shoppers, blurts, "I seek God! I seek God!" "The madman jumped into their midst and pierced them with his eyes," Nietzsche continues. "'Whither is God?' he cried; 'I will tell you. *We have killed him*—you and I. All of us are his murderers. . . . God is dead. God remains dead. And we have killed him'" (Nietzsche, 1974, 181).

Nietzsche's announcement of the death of God has been interpreted in many ways: as an affront to Christianity, a declaration of anarchy, or nihilism of the most dangerous kind. But careful readers know that there is much more to the story than this. What Nietzsche was proclaiming is that given the skepticism of scientific inquiry, the technologies birthed by it, and their globalizing, industrializing, and militarizing effects, Europeans were finding it increasingly difficult to believe in anything with transcendent value. By the end of the nineteenth century, in other words, God had "died" to the experience of the average

European. Their once-enchanted world had been supplanted by a mechanistic universe, in which they were little more than expendable cogs.

Mechanistic philosophy sees the body as a system of brute matter capable of being observed, measured, and controlled. Stripped of any connection to the gods and/or to any ultimate significance, human life becomes a matter of the *Körper*: a quantifiable, de-animated substance that can be managed like water, air, and crops, according to objective calculative procedures. Liberals, conservatives, Marxists, and fascists alike all endorse variations of this idea. (Self-proclaimed futurist, Filippo Marinetti, for example, does so in his aesthetics of the synchronized goosestep, where he envisions the "metalization of the human body.") For it promises total mastery over the instability and precariousness of nature, including *human* nature. In the case of biomedicine in particular, this mechanistic worldview holds out the promise of an end to disease, bodily decrepitude, and, ultimately, death itself.

Driven by the progress of the natural sciences, by the end of the nineteenth century it appeared to many commentators that humanity was at last on the cusp of fulfilling the ancient prophecy that "Ye shall be as gods!" (Fromm, 1966). Yet already suspicions both about the plausibility and the wisdom of this mechanistic picture were being aired by those (sometimes derisively) called "Romantics." Every nation had them. There were the English poets William Blake, William Wordsworth, and Samuel Coleridge; their American counterparts Ralph Waldo Emerson and Henry David Thoreau; the French essayist Jean Jacques Rousseau, as well as Charles Baudelaire and Jean Rimbaud. However much their cautions were tinctured by their unique backgrounds, all of them expressed apprehension about the social transformations they were witnessing. They decried how these devalued nature, belittled the creative spontaneity of bodily instincts, denigrated human desire, and overlooked the emotional storms and stresses of real life.

Romanticism flourished in intellectual circles throughout Europe, but its most decisive impact was in Germany. One reason for this is that the petty German kingdoms of the early nineteenth century were on the receiving end of Napoléon Bonaparte's designs to remake Europe after the presumed universal principles of French *civilité*. A second, more important, reason was resentment over the imposition of Prussian bureaucracy on the rest of the German states after 1870. In an effort to advertise their singularity both from the considered drab conventions of bourgeois France on the one hand and the "polar night of icy darkness and hardness" (as Max Weber describes Prussian domination [1946, 128]) on the other, German Romantics residing in Bavaria and Badenia began to extol the themes of Dionysian warmth and unfettered eroticism. In doing so, they drew on a deep current of Christian mysticism traceable at least back to Meister Eckhart and John Tauler.

During the nineteenth century, the German landscape underwent profound alterations. In 1800, the country had only twenty-two million inhabitants. Within one hundred years it could boast of housing nearly three times that number, the largest population on the continent. Most of these lived in places other than where they had been born, in burgeoning commercial centers. By 1910, Germany had as many large cities as all of the rest of Europe combined, and it had overtaken both England and France as a military power. One American studying in Germany in 1870—for Germany by now had also become the world's leader in graduate education and research—described the grand entrance of the *Wehrmacht* into Berlin after its victory over the French army at Sedan earlier that year: "It was the most magnificent manifestation of power that the world has ever furnished" (Burgess, 1966, 96). Perhaps most tellingly, by 1900 an estimated one-tenth of the German labor force was comprised of private or public bureaucrats, nearly ten times the number of those employed in "free" nonagricultural jobs. In short, in less than three generations, the rustic German *Gemeinschaften* (communities), whose kin were united on the basis of their attachment to shared blood and soil, had been superseded by impersonal *Gesellschaften* (corporate associations) comprised of self-interested egos whose obligations to each other were limited to formal job descriptions and contracts (Tönnies, 1957). To quote Weber, the Fatherland had evolved into an "iron cage" inhabited by "specialists without spirit, sensualists without heart; [a] nullity [that] imagines . . . it has attained a level of civilization never before achieved" (Weber, 1958, 181–82).

Martin Heidegger writes of historical ruptures that occur in a "flashing glance" (*Augenblich*), when the calcified assumptions of an old lifeworld collapse and a clearing is created for the possibility of new musical, artistic, poetic, and dramatic insights. The emergence of the nineteenth-century German Romantics documents just such a moment. As German society was becoming increasingly regimented according to machine specifications, and its military was reaching deadly heights, life (*Leben*) began to reveal itself. This was not life in the scientific sense—the quantifiable functioning of organisms as discerned by controlled experimentation—but the sensual, historically situated movement of vital existence.

Lebensphilosophie

In protest against the leveling down of all things to the observable motions of de-animated matter, German Romantics began extolling *Lebensphilosophie* (life philosophy). Its goal would be to artistically, poetically, and dramatically recapture life *as it is lived*; a phenomenon so complex, nuanced, and dynamic as be to incapable of being compartmentalized, counted, and weighed like objective facts. Life is beyond scientific analysis, argued the proponents of *Lebensphilosophie*, because science itself *is* a living act. Without life there can be no science.

Lebensphilosophie led to a number of developments, some of them laughable, others tragic. One of its more innocent manifestations was the pacifist, alcohol-abstinent back-to-nature youth movement (*Wandervögel* = wandering bird), whose members hiked together and camped out. Its more radical followers advocated nudism (*blosses Leben* = naked life) and, in response to the advent of socialized (bureaucratized) medicine by Otto Bismarck in 1884, natural healing. The *Wandervögel* abjured notions of timid, stuffy citified customs, opting instead to don the colorful dress of the peasantry and to commune with the forest. Some observers believe it to have been the historical precursor of the flower-bedecked American hippie movement of the late 1960s (Kennedy, 1998).

In England, *Lebensphilosophie* found voice in the writings of D. H. Lawrence, who received it directly via his adulterous affair with Frieda von Richthofen (Green, 1974). Lawrence's classic novel, *Lady Chatterley's Lover*, unfavorably contrasts the prosperous estate owner, Clifford, "shipped home smashed" and impotent from World War I with his primitive, sexually virile gamekeeper, Mellors, who steals Clifford's wife's affections. Clifford represents to Lawrence high bourgeois England, which glories in its technological prowess and its devotion to the staid class system. Mellors signifies the irrepressible chthonic force of life that shatters its pretensions.

A second, more frightening, development out of *Lebensphilosophie* was its nazification by principled anti-intellectuals such as Ludwig Klages and Alfred Baeumler. To Klages and Baeumler the purpose of thinking is not, as the Socratic tradition teaches, to discern fixed principles. The reason for this is that there are none. There is only the flux and flow of life. One's duty therefore is not to resist life's vital impulses, but to surrender to them, enjoying their bounty. Nor is the task of history to painstakingly depict the development of belief systems using the methods of positivist historiography. Instead, it is to prepare readers for "open war" against the forces of cold ("Jewish") empirical reason, "mythify" history, and offer compelling, if fanciful, accounts of the Greco-Teutonic past. When done well, Klages and Baeumler claimed, such accounts would evoke in audiences the intoxicating ecstasy, the *Rausch* (rush), of communal remembrance (Lebovic, 2006).

Klages and Baeumler depicted the agonies of life, the struggles that arise from the unconscious desires of flesh, from soul-craving, and the yearning for freedom. At the same time, they denounced German militarism and colonialism, which they considered Machiavellian expressions of instrumental logic. The subtlety of this distinction would be lost when Klages and Baeumler were appropriated and vulgarized by Nazi propaganda minister, Alfred Rosenberg, and rendered into the kinds of vicious images familiar to readers today.

Philosopher Wilhelm Dilthey represents a third, considerably more palatable, manifestation of *Lebensphilosophie*. In his hands it led to a new way to do history. The goal of what Dilthey called *Geisteswissenschaft* (*Geist* = spirit [culture] + *Wissenschaft* = science) is not to causally *explain* why things happened in the past, but to aid audiences to understand (*Verstehen*) them, to place readers in the historical subject's shoes so that they might access that subject's reality (Dilthey, 1961). This requires historians to "psychologically enter" into the events and people they study, instead of observing them from a distance—unearthing the lived experience (*Erlebnis*) lying behind their legends and rites.

Geisteswissenschaften would eventually evolve into the practice of modern ethnography. It would also serve as an indirect inspiration for Martin Heidegger's approach to phenomenology. Heidegger, however, rejected the Diltheyian program because of what he believed was its unacceptably casual, "ambiguous," and "hazy" use of the term "life" (Heidegger, 2001b, 62). For Heidegger, phenomenology could never achieve, as Dilthey had hoped, a definitively accurate and complete account of life. On the contrary, the most that can be expected from it are "provisional" or "indicative" (*anzeigen*) aspects of lived experience. These might disclose some facets of how people exist, but only at the price of hiding others. For Heidegger, to reveal is to conceal; seeing things one way is to be blinded to others.

Following Nietzsche's path, Heidegger went on to undermine the legitimacy of the core assumptions of European philosophy and science. He did this by critiquing its urge to discover a ground for certain knowledge. Heidegger believed that the desire for unassailable truth has, over the centuries, diverted philosophy from the *actual* "thing itself," which, for him, is the inherent uncertainty and precariousness of life. By "fleeing in the face of [life's eerie contingency and instability]," traditional philosophy and science "misplaces and disguises" life (Heidegger, 2001b, 81). In the hands of philosophy and science, life becomes just another object, an obstacle to be instrumentally managed.

Phenomenology

The grand hopes for a society founded on the revolutionary principles of *liberté, egalité,* and *fraternité* culminated in the French "Reign of Terror" of 1789. This was a powerful spur for the Romantic revolt against instrumental rationality. World War I (1914–1918) had a similar dispiriting effect. And if the mud-trench horror of this, the "war to end all wars," was not enough to convince witnesses of the hollowness of the dream of scientifically engineered progress, then certainly the industrialized death camps of World War II supplied it. With the ghostly specter of murdered millions haunting the intellectual scene during the twentieth century, *Lebensphilosophie* and phenomenology began to gain purchase outside Germany. For six years (1933–1939), Russian émigré Alexandre Kojève conducted philosophy seminars in Paris at the École Practique des Hautes Études. There he introduced Heidegger to a group of young French thinkers, including Jacques Lacan, Georges Bataille, Maurice Merleau-Ponty, Eric Weil, and André Breton, all of whom had already become disillusioned with the rigid, archaic French academic system. And following his stay in Berlin in the early 1930s, Jean-Paul Sartre popularized Heidegger's *Being and Time* in his own *Being and Nothingness*. French philosophy would never be the same (Kleinberg, 2005).

Something comparable occurred in American intellectual circles. It was American physicists who manufactured the A-bomb; American cold warriors who devised the logic of MAD-ness (mutually assured destruction) to deter its use against themselves. Thus, not even the New World could remain oblivious to the dimming prospects for progress after 1950. While the popular response to this sobering realization was a virulent brand of anti-intellectual, isolationist Christian fundamentalism, in academia it created an audience receptive to phenomenology. Heidegger and his protégés as a result began to find a home in the United States, carried to America largely by émigrés fleeing Nazi repression. By 1958 the first accessible introduction to existential phenomenology had been authored by the philosopher William

Barrett (1962). Since that time phenomenology has firmly rooted itself in the humanities professorate along both coasts, and is at this writing penetrating the social sciences (most notably, sociology and anthropology), as well as pedagogy and the "helping professions": social work, physical therapy, and nursing.

In the course of these developments, a basic theme endures, namely, skepticism concerning "scientism," where science is dogmatically accepted as the only method to obtain truth (Heidegger, 2001a, 18). As Nietzsche proclaimed through the voice of his fictional madman, scientism has resulted in God's "death." Or, to use Heidegger's expression, scientism has severed the event of life from its connection to earth, and living beings from their ties to each other. As Heidegger wrote in 1935:

> The spiritual decline of the earth has progressed so far that peoples are in danger of losing their last spiritual strength, the strength that makes it possible even to see the decline and to appraise it as such. This simple observation has nothing to do with cultural pessimism—nor with any optimism either, of course; for the darkening of the world, the flight of the gods, the destruction of the earth, the reduction of human beings to a mass, the hatred and mistrust of everything creative and free has already reached such proportions throughout the whole earth that such childish categories as pessimism and optimism have long become laughable. (2000, 40)

His own controversial alliance with Nazism aside, Heidegger's words speak to today's generation. They remind us that lurking just beneath the floor of the iron (and now silicon) cage in which we all scurry about lies a mysterious "happening" (*Geschehen*), the happening of life. The more frantically we flee it, the more we treat it as an object to be fixed and corrected (i.e., "made right") by technical procedures, the more we are destined to suffer the anxiety of "not being at home" (*Unheimlichkeit*).

References

Acocella, J. (1998, April 9). The Politics of Hysteria. *The New Yorker*, 64–79.

Agger, B. (2004). *Speeding Up Fast Capitalism*. Boulder, CO: Paradigm Pub.

Agger, B., and B. Shelton. (2007). *Fast Families, Virtual Children*. Boulder, CO: Paradigm Pub.

Aho, J. (2002). *The Orifice As Sacrificial Site*. Hawthorne, NY: Aldine DeGruyter.

———. (2005). *Confession and Bookkeeping*. Albany, NY: SUNY Press.

Aho, K. (2007). Acceleration and Time Pathologies: The Critique of Psychology in Heidegger's Beiträge. *Time and Society*, *16*, 25–42.

Alcoholics Anonymous. (2002). *The Big Book*. N.p.: AA World Services, Inc.

Anderson, J. A. (2001). Awaiting Demands of Tomorrow's Patients. Retrieved from the World Wide Web: www.Amednews.com.

Anderson, T. C. (1997). Technology and the Decline of Leisure. *Proceedings of the American Catholic Philosophical Association*, *7*, 1–15.

Anonymous. (1956). *The Pittsburgh Trial*. Wichita, KS: Defender Publishers.

Anspach, R. (1994). The Language of Case Presentation. In P. Conrad and R. Kern (eds.), *The Sociology of Health and Illness*. Fourth edition. New York: St. Martin's Press.

Appleton, N. (1999). *The Curse of Louis Pasteur*. N.p.: Choice Pub.

Arabella. (n.d.). The Mysterious Zār. Retrieved from the World Wide Web: www.Shira.net/arabella/zar.html.

Ash, P. (1949). The Reliability of Psychiatric Diagnosis. *Journal of Abnormal and Social Psychology*, *44*, 272–76.

Associated Press. (2007, October 12). Is Rise in Bipolar Kids Real? *Idaho State Journal*.

Aylett, R. (2002). *Robots: Bringing Intelligent Machines to Life?* Hauppage, NY: Quarto Pub.

Bakalar, N. (2003). *Where the Germs Are*. Hoboken, NJ: John Wiley.

Baker, A. (1994). *Awakening Our Self-Healing Body*. La Jolla, CA: Self-Health Care Systems.

Balch, P. (2006). *Prescription for Nutritional Health*. Fourth edition. Garden City, NY: Avery Pub.

Baldry, P. E. (1976 [1965]). *The Battle Against Bacteria*. London: Cambridge University Press.

Banks, A. (1999). *Birth, Chairs, Midwives, and Medicine*. Jackson: University Press of Mississippi.

Barker, K. (2002). Self-Help Literature and the Making of an Illness Identity: The Case of Fibromyalgia. *Social Problems, 49*, 279–300.

Barrett, W. (1962). *Irrational Man*. New York: Vintage Books.

Barsky, A. J., and J. F. Borus. (1999). Functional Somatic Syndromes. *Annals of Internal Medicine, 130*, 910–21.

Bass, W., and J. Jefferson. (2004). *Death's Acre: Inside the Legendary Forensics Lab the Body Farm*. New York: Berkeley.

Bates, M., W. T. Edwards, and K. Anderson. (1993). Ethnocultural Influences on Variation in Chronic Pain Perception. *Pain, 52*, 101–12.

Beard, G. M. (1880). *A Practical Treatise on Nervous Exhaustion (Neurasthenia): Its Symptoms, Nature*. New York: Wood.

Beardon, T. (n.d.). Royal Raymond Rife. Retrieved from the World Wide Web: www.Cheniere.org/books/aids/rife.

Becker, E. (1973). *The Denial of Death*. New York: Free Press

———. (1975). *Escape from Evil*. New York: Free Press.

———. (2005). Social Science and Psychiatry. In D. Liechty (ed.), *The Ernest Becker Reader*. Seattle: University of Washington Press.

Bedell, S. E., T. B. Graboys, E. Bedell, and B. Lown. (2004). Words that Harm, Words that Heal. *Archives of Internal Medicine, 164*, 1365–67.

Bell, S. (1990). Changing Ideas: The Medicalization of Menopause. In R. Romaner (ed.), *Meanings of Menopause*. Hillsdale, NJ: Analytic Press.

Berger, P. (1969). *The Sacred Canopy*. New York: Doubleday-Anchor.

Berger, P., and T. Luckmann. (1967). *The Social Construction of Reality*. Garden City, NY: Doubleday Anchor.

Bertman, S. (1998). *Hyperculture: The Human Cost of Speed*. Westport, CT: Praeger Publishers.

Best, J. (ed.). (1989). *Images of Issues*. First edition. Hawthorne, NY: Aldine de Gruyter.

———. (ed.). (1995). *Images of Issues*. Second edition. Hawthorne, NY: Aldine de Gruyter.

Binswanger, L. (1956). Existential Analysis and Psychotherapy. In Fromm, Reichman and Moreno (eds.), *Progress in Psychotherapy*. New York: Grune and Stratton.

Bird, C. (1991). *The Persecution and Trial of Gaston Naessens*. Tiburon, CA: H. J. Kramer, Inc.

———. (n.da.). Royal R. Rife. Retrieved from the World Wide Web: www.navi.net~rsc/rife1.

———. (n.db.). The Mystery of Pleomorphic Microbial Organisms. Retrieved from the World Wide Web: www.whale.to/p/bird.

Bizzari, H. F. (n.d.). The Zār Ceremony. Retrieved from the World Wide Web: www.touregypt.net/featurestories/zar.html.

Boddy, C. (1989). *Wombs and Alien Spirits*. Madison: Wisconsin University Press.

Bourdieu, P. (1963). The Attitude of the Algerian Peasant toward Time. In J. Pitt-Rivers (ed.), *Mediterranean Countrymen*. Paris: Mouton.

Bracken, P., and P. Thomas. (2005). *Postpsychiatry: Mental Health in the Postmodern World*. New York: Oxford University Press.

Brown, P., S. Zavestoski, S. McCormick, M. Linder, J. Mandelbaum, and T. Luebke. (2000). A Gulf of Difference: Disputes over Gulf War-Related Illnesses. *Journal of Health and Social Behavior, 42*, 235–57.

Brown, T. (1985). Descartes, Dualism, and Psychosomatic Medicine. In W. F. Bynum et al. (eds.), *The Anatomy of Madness*. London: Tavistock.

Bruce, D. (2003). *Miracle Touch*. New York: Three Rivers Press.

Bunce, J. (2006). Parasite "Turns Women into Sex Kittens." Retrieved from the World Wide Web: www.news.com.au.

Burgess, J. (1966). *Reminiscences of an American Scholar*. New York: AMS Press.

C. A. K. (1934). Hume, E. Douglas, "Béchamp or Pasteur?" *Isis, 21*, 404–5.

Callihan, D. (1995). Through the Window of Pain. Retrieved from the World Wide Web: www.umc.pitt.edu/pittmag/sep95/painh.

Calvin, J. (1956). *On God and Man* (F. W. Strothmann, ed.). New York: Frederick Ungar.

Campo, R. (2003). *The Healing Art*. New York: W.W. Norton.

Camus, A. (1946). *The Stranger* (S. Gilbert, trans.). New York: Vintage Books.

Carman, T. (1999). The Body in Husserl and Merleau-Ponty. *Philosophical Topics, 27*, 205–26.

Carter, R. (1983). *Descartes' Medical Philosophy: The Organic Solution to the Mind-Body Problem*. Baltimore: Johns Hopkins University Press.

Cassell, E. (1976). Illness and Disease. *Hastings Center Report, 6*, 27–37.

———. (1991). *The Nature of Suffering and the Goals of Medicine*. New York: Oxford University Press.

Cerbone, D. (2000). Heidegger and Dasein's Bodily Nature: What is the Hidden Problematic? *International Journal of Philosophical Studies, 9*, 209–30.

Cheng, Y., L. Ching-Polin, H. Lu, Y. Hsu, L. Kun-Eng, D. Hung, et al. (2007). Expertise Modulates in the Perception of Pain in Others. *Current Biology, 17*, 1708–13.

Chesterton, G. K. (1959 [1908]). The Ethics of Elfland. In G. K. Chesterton (ed.), *Orthodoxy*. Garden City, NY: Image Books.

Chin, T. (2003). Lurking, Listening, Learning: Using Online Support Groups. Retrieved from the World Wide Web: www.Amednews.com.

Chodoff, P. (2002). The Medicalization of the Human Condition. *Psychiatric Services, 53*, 627–28.

Cooley, C. H. (1902). *Human Nature and Social Order*. New York: Charles Scribner's Sons.

Corea, G. (1986). *The Mother Machine: Reproductive Technologies from Artificial Insemination to Artificial Wombs.* New York: Harper and Row.

Crain, C. (1999, August). Did A Germ Make You Gay? *Out,* 46–49.

Cushman, P. (2003). How Psychology Erodes Personhood. *Journal of Theoretical and Philosophical Psychology, 22,* 103–13.

Cushman, P., and P. Gilford. (2000). Will Managed Care Change our Way of Being? *American Psychologist, 55,* 985–96.

Damasio, A. (1999). *The Feeling of What Happens: Body and Emotion in the Making of Consciousness.* New York: Harcourt and Brace.

Davis-Floyd, R., and J. Dumit (eds.). (1998). *Cyborg Babies: From Techno-Sex to Techno-Tots.* New York: Routledge.

De Kruif, P. (1959 [1926]). *The Microbe Hunters.* New York: Pocket Books.

DeMets, D. L., and T. R. Fleming. (1996). Surrogate End Points in Clinical Trials: Are We Being Misled? *Annals of Internal Medicine, 125,* 605–13.

Denzinger, H. (ed.). (1957). *The Sources of Catholic Dogma* (R. Deferrari, trans.). St. Louis: Herder.

DeRubeis, R. J., L. A. Gelfand, T. Z. Tang, and A. D. Simons. (1999). Medications Versus Cognitive Behavior Therapy for Severely Depressed Outpatients. *American Journal of Psychiatry, 156,* 1007–25.

Dilthey, W. (1961). *Pattern and Meaning in History* (H. Rickman, ed.). New York: Harper & Row.

Dimidjian, S., K. S. Dobson, R. J. Kohlenberg, R. Gallop, D. K. Markley, D. C. Atkins, et al. (2006). Randomized Trial of Behavioral Activation, Cognitive Therapy, and Antidepressant Medication in the Acute Treatment of Adults with Major Depression. *Journal of Consulting and Clinical Psychology, 74,* 658–70.

Donohoe, M. (2006). Beauty and Body Modification. Retrieved from the World Wide Web: www.medscape.com/viewarticle/529442.

Dossey, L. (1993). *Healing Words: The Power of Prayer and the Practice of Medicine.* New York: HarperCollins.

Dresden, E. H. (June 7, 1931). Germs, the Modern Superstition. *Golden Age,* 404–6.

Dubos, R. (1994 [1960]). *Pasteur and Modern Science.* Washington, DC: AMS Press.

Duclaux, E. (1920). *Pasteur: The History of a Mind* (E. Smith and F. Hedges, trans.). Philadelphia: W. B. Saunders.

Ehrenreich, B., and D. English. (2005). *For Her Own Good.* Second edition. New York: Anchor Books.

Eisenberg, D. M., R. C. Kesseler, C. Foster, F. E. Norlock, D. R. Calkins, and T. L. Delbanco. (1993). Unconventional Medicine in the United States. *New England Journal of Medicine, 238,* 246–52.

Elias, M. (2002, March 8). Friends May Make Breast Cancer More Survivable. *USA Today.*

Elliot, C. (2008, January 7). Guinea-Pigging. *The New Yorker,* 36–41.

Engel, G. (1977). The Need for A New Medical Model: A Challenge for Biomedicine. *Science, 196,* 29–136.

———. (1980). The Clinical Application of the Biopsychosocial Model. *American Journal of Psychiatry, 137*, 535–44.

Erchak, G., and R. Rosenfeld. (1989). Learning Disabilities, Dyslexia, and the Medicalization of the Classroom. In J. Best (ed.), *Images of Issues*. Hawthorne, NY: Aldine de Gruyter.

Evernden, N. (1992). *The Social Creation of Nature*. Baltimore: Johns Hopkins University Press.

Feinstein, A. (1983). An Additional Basic Science for Clinical Measurement. *Annals of Internal Medicine, 99*, 705–12.

Fischoff, B., and S. Wesseley. (2003). Managing Patients with Inexplicable Health Problems. *British Medical Journal, 3*, 282–84.

Florine, Hans. (n.d.). Hans Florine. Retrieved from the World Wide Web: www.hansflorine.com.

Foucault, M. (1965). *Madness and Civilization: A History of Insanity in the Age of Reason* (A. M. S. Smith, trans.). New York: Random House.

———. (1975). *The Birth of the Clinic: An Archaeology of Medical Perception* (A. M. S. Smith, trans.). New York: Vintage Books.

———. (1990 [1978]). *The History of Sexuality* (R. Hurley, trans.). New York: Pantheon.

Freidman, M., and R. H. Rosenman. (1959). Association of Specific Overt Behavior Patterns with Blood and Cardiovascular Findings. *JAMA, 161*, 1286–96.

Freud, S. (1962). *Civilization and Its Discontents* (J. Strachey, trans.). New York: W.W. Norton.

Freud, S., and J. Breuer. (1952). *Studies in Hysteria*. New York: Penguin Books.

Freund, P., M. McGuire, and L. Podhurst. (2003). *Health, Illness, and the Social Body*. Upper Saddle River, NJ: Prentice-Hall.

Fromm, E. (1966). *Ye Shall Be As Gods*. New York: Holt, Rinehart & Winston.

Fuchs, T. (2003). The Phenomenology of Shame, Guilt and the Body in Body Dysmorphic Disorder and Depression. *Journal of Phenomenological Psychiatry, 33*, 223–43.

———. (2005). Corporealized and Disembodied Minds: A Phenomenological View of the Body in Melancholia and Schizophrenia. *Philosophy, Psychiatry, and Psychology, 12*, 95–107.

———. (n.d.). The Phenomenology of the Body and Space in Depression. Retrieved from the World Wide Web: www.inet.uni2.dk/home/ifpl (private).

Gadamer, H. G. (1994). *Truth and Method* (J. Weinsheimer and D. Marshall, trans.). New York: Continuum Press.

———. (1996). *The Enigma of Health*. Stanford, CA: Stanford University Press.

Geison, G. (1995). *The Private Science of Louis Pasteur*. Princeton, NJ: Princeton University Press.

Gilman, S., H. King, R. Porter, G. S. Rousseau, and E. Showalter. (1993). *Hysteria Beyond Freud*. Berkeley: University of California Press.

Gladwell, M. (1999, February 15). Running from Ritalin. *The New Yorker*, 80–84.

Gleick, J. (2000). *Faster: The Acceleration of Practically Everything*. New York: Pantheon.

Goffman, E. (1959). *The Presentation of Self in Everyday Life*. New York: Doubleday-Anchor.

———. (1963). *Stigma: Notes on the Management of Spoiled Identity*. New York: Touchstone Books.

Goldberg, M. (2007). *Kingdom Coming*. New York: W.W. Norton.

Goodman, E. (1998, July 14). Silicone Misuse Not Science's Fault. *Idaho State Journal*.

Greco, M. (1998). *Illness As A Work of Thought*. New York: Routledge.

Green, M. (1974). *The Von Richthofen Sisters*. Albuquerque: University of New Mexico Press.

Greenberg, G. (2007, May). Manufacturing Depression. *Harper's Magazine*, 35–47.

Grohol, J. (n.d.). Teen Homicide, Suicide, and Firearm Death. Retrieved from the World Wide Web: www.childtrendsdatabank.org/indicators/70ViolentDeath.cfm.

Groopman, J. (2000, November). Hurting All Over, *The New Yorker*, 78–88.

———. (2001, December 3). Eyes Wide Open. *The New Yorker*, 52–57.

———. (2007, January 29). What's the Trouble? *The New Yorker*, 36–41.

Guignon, C. (1983). *Heidegger and the Problem of Knowledge*. Indianapolis: Hackett Press.

———. (2002). Hermeneutics, Authenticity, and the Aims of Psychology. *Journal of Theoretical and Philosophical Psychology*, 22, 83–102.

Guterman, L. (2005, December 2). Duping the Brain into Healing the Body. *Chronicle of Higher Education*, A-12 to A-14.

Hancock, L. (1995, March 6). Breaking Point. *Newsweek*, 56–61.

Haraway, D. (1991). A Cyborg Manifesto: Science, Technology, and Socialist-Feminism in the Late Twentieth Century. In D. Haraway (ed.), *Simians, Cyborgs and Women*. New York: Routledge.

Harder, B. (2006, September 2). Sleep Treatments Rise to the Occasion. *USA Today*.

Harris, G. (2006, November 23). Proof is Scant on Psychiatric Drug Mix for Young. *New York Times*.

Harris, G., and J. Roberts. (2007, March 21). Doctors' Ties to Drug Makers Are Put on Close View. *New York Times*.

Hassett, A. L., and L. H. Sigal. (2002). Unforeseen Consequences of Terrorism. *Archives of Internal Medicine*, 162, 1809–13.

Hearn, G. (2006). Physicians and Functional Syndromes: No Clue—Many Opinions. Unpublished paper presented to annual meeting of the American Sociological Association, Montreal, Canada.

Heidegger, M. (1962). *Being and Time* (J. Maccquarrie and E. Robinson, trans.). New York: Harper & Row.

———. (1977a). *The Question Concerning Technology* (W. Lovitt, trans.). New York: Harper & Row.

———. (1977b). Letter on Humanism (A. Hofstadter, trans.). In D. Krell (ed.), *Basic Writings*. San Francisco: HarperCollins

———. (1977c). What is Metaphysics? (A. Hofstadter, trans.). In D. Krell (ed.), *Basic Writings*. San Francisco: HarperCollins.

———. (1977d). Building, Dwelling, Thinking (A. Hofstadter, trans.). In D. Krell (ed.), *BasicWritings*. San Francisco: HarperCollins.

———. (1982). *Basic Problems of Phenomenology* (A. Hofstadter, trans.). Bloomington: Indiana University Press.

———. (1985). *The History of the Concept of Time* (Theodore Kisiel, trans.). Bloomington: Indiana University Press.

———. (1992). *The Concept of Time* (W. McNeill, trans.). Oxford, England: Blackwell.

———. (1995). *The Fundamental Concepts of Metaphysics* (W. McNeill and N. Walker, trans.). Bloomington: Indiana University Press.

———. (1999). *Contributions to Philosophy (From Enowning)* (P. Emad and K. Maly, trans.). Bloomington: Indiana University Press.

———. (2000). *Introduction to Metaphysics* (G. Fried and R. Polt, trans.). New Haven, CT: Yale University Press.

———. (2001a). *Zollikon Seminars* (F. Mayr and R. Askay, trans.). Evanston, IL: Northwestern University Press.

———. (2001b). *Phenomenological Interpretations of Aristotle* (R. Wojcewicz, trans.). Bloomington: Indiana University Press.

———. (2005). *Introduction to Phenomenological Research* (D. Dahlstrom, trans.). Bloomington: Indiana University Press.

Hempel, C. (1966). *Philosophy of Natural Science*. Englewood, NJ: Prentice-Hall.

Hewitt, J. (1991). *Self & Society*. Fifth edition. Boston: Allyn & Bacon.

Hirshbein, L. (2006). Science, Gender, and the Emergence of Depression in American Psychiatry, 1952–1980. *Journal of the History of Medicine, 61*, 187–216.

Hochschild, A. (1983). *The Managed Heart: The Commercialization of Emotion*. Berkeley: University of California Press.

Hopper, J. (1999). The New Germ Theory. *Atlantic Monthly, 283*, 41–50.

Horrobin, D. (n.d.). *Medical Hubris: A Reply to Ivan Illich*. Montreal, Canada: Eden Press.

House, J., K. Landis, and D. Umberson. (1994). Social Relations and Health. In P. Conrad and R. Kern (eds.), *The Sociology of Health & Illness*. Fourth edition. New York: St. Martin's Press.

Hoxsey, H. (1956). *You Don't Have to Die*. New York: Milestone Books, Inc.

Hughes, J. A. (2003, December 1). While Medicine Caters to Spoiled Patients, the Truly Ill Go Wanting. *American Medical News*.

Hunt, W. (1976, May 6). The Persecution of H. Ray Evers, M.D. *National Chronicle*.

Hurst, J. W. (2003). What Do Good Doctors Try to Do? *Archives of Internal Medicine, 163*, 2681–86.

Husserl, E. (1970). *The Crisis of European Science* (D. Carr, trans.). Evanston, IL: Northwestern University Press.

———. (1977). *The Cartesian Meditations: An Introduction to Phenomenology* (D. Cairns, trans.). The Hague: Martinus Nijhoff.

———. (1996). Phenomenology. In R. Kearney and M. Rainwater (eds), *The Continental Philosophy Reader*. London and New York: Routledge.

Illich, I. (1976). *Limits to Medicine. Medical Nemesis: The Expropriation of Health.* New York: Pantheon Books.

Iwado, Z. T. (1937). Hagakure Bushido (The Book of the Warrior). *Cultural Nippon, 7,* 33–55.

Jewson, N. D. (1976). The Disappearance of the Sick-Man from Medical Cosmology, 1770–1870. *Sociology, 10,* 225–44.

Johnson, J. (1989). Horror Stories and the Construction of Child Abuse. In J. Best (ed), *Images of Issues*. Hawthorne, NY: Aldine de Gruyter.

Jonas, H. (1966). *The Phenomenon of Life*. New York: Harper & Row.

Kabat-Zinn, J. (1990). *Full Catastrophe Living*. New York: Delta Books.

Katz, J. (1995). *The Invention of Heterosexuality*. New York: Penguin Books.

Kennedy, G. (1998). *Children of the Sun*. N.p.: Nirvana Press.

Kern, S. (1983). *The Culture of Time and Space: 1880–1918*. Cambridge, MA: Harvard University Press.

Kleinberg, E. (2005). *Generation Existential: Heidegger's Philosophy in France, 1927–1961*. Ithaca, NY: Cornell University Press.

Kleinman, A. (1988). *The Illness Narratives: Suffering, Healing and the Human Condition*. New York: Basic Books.

Klevins, R. M., M. A. Morrison, J. Nadle, S. Petit, K. Gershman, S. Ray, et al. (2007). Invasive Methicillin-Resistant *Staphylococcus Aureus* Infections in the United States. *JAMA, 298,* 1763–71.

Kolata, G. (1994, October 21). Study Says 1 in 5 Americans Suffers from Chronic Pain. *New York Times*.

Kos Pharmaceuticals. (2006). Niaspan (R) Combined with Low/Moderate Dosed Statin Achieves Better Total Lipid Control. Retrieved from the World Wide Web: Today.Reuters.com/stocks/quoteCompanyNewsArticle.aspx?view=pr&symbol=kosp.o.

Kramer, P. (1997). *Listening to Prozac: Remaking the Self in the Age of Antidepressants*. New York: Penguin.

———. (2006, August 30). Is Everybody Happy? An Interview with "Listening to Prozac" Author. Retrieved from the World Wide Web: www.psychology today.com/articles/pto-20011101-000031.html.

Krieg, E. (2000). Therapeutic Touch: Does it Work? Retrieved from the World Wide Web: www.PhACT.org/e/tt.

Kroll-Smith, S., and H. Floyd. (1997). *Bodies in Protest*. New York: New York University Press.

Kuczynski, A. (2006). *Beauty Junkies*. New York: Doubleday Books.

Kuhn, R. (1976). *The Demon of Noontide: Ennui in Western Literature*. Princeton, NJ: Princeton University Press.

Kuhn, T. (1970). *The Structure of Scientific Revolution*. Second edition (enl). Chicago: University of Chicago Press.

Küspert, G. (2006). *Streitpunkt: Krankheit. Die Kontroverse um Funktionelle Syndrome Zwischen Medizineurn und Laien in den USA*. Inaugural dissertation. Erlangen—Nürmberg: Friedrich Alexander Universität.

Kutchins, H., and S. Kirk. (1997). *Making Us Crazy: DSM, The Psychiatric Bible and the Creation of Mental Disorders*. New York: Free Press.

Lazarou, J., B. H. Pomeranz, and P. N. Corey. (1998). Incidence of Adverse Drug Reactions in Hospitalized Patients. *JAMA, 279*, 1200–1205.

Lebovic, N. (2006). The Beauty and Terror of Lebensphilosophie. *South Central Review, 23*, 23–39.

Lederer, W. (1968). *The Fear of Women*. New York: Harcourt Brace Jovanovich.

Lefkowitz, M. (1996, February 26–March 4). The Wandering Womb. *The New Yorker*, 94.

Lerner, Barron. (2006). *When Illness Goes Public*. Baltimore: Johns Hopkins University Press.

Lester, D. (1972). Voodoo Death. *American Anthropologist, 74*, 386–90.

Levine, B. (2001). *A Review of Commonsense Rebellion*. N.p.: Continuum Pub. Group, Inc.

Levine, R. (1997). *A Geography of Time*. New York: Basic Books.

———. (2005). A Geography of Busyness, *Social Research, 72*, 355–70.

Levine, S. (1989). *Healing into Life and Death*. New York: Anchor.

Lewis, B. (2002). *What Went Wrong?* New York: Harper Perennial.

Liberman, J. (1990). *Light: Medicine of the Future*. N.p.: Bear & Co.

Livingston, K. (1997). Ritalin: Miracle Drug or Cop-Out? *The Public Interest, 127*, 3–18.

Loy, D. (1996). *Lack and Transcendence: The Problem of Death and Life in Psychotherapy, Existentialism, and Buddhism*. New York: Prometheus.

———. (2002). *A Buddhist History of the West*. Albany, NY: SUNY Press.

Lumley, M., L. Stettner, and F. Wehmer. (1996). How are Alexithymia and Physical Illness Linked? A Review and Critique of Pathways. *Journal of Psychosomatic Research, 41*, 505–18.

Lutz, T. (1991). *American Nervousness, 1903: An Anecdotal History*. Ithaca, NY: Cornell University Press.

Maines, R. (1999). *The Technology of Orgasm*. Baltimore: Johns Hopkins University Press.

Malleson, A. (2002). *Whiplash and Other Useful Illnesses*. Montreal, Canada: McGill-Queen's University Press.

Mander, J. (1991). *In the Absence of the Sacred*. San Francisco: Sierra Club Books.

Markle, C. E., and F. B. McCrea. (2008). *What if Medicine Disappeared?* Albany, NY: SUNY Press.

Martinez, R. (2003). Scenario: How Do You Manage Challenging Encounters? Retrieved from the World Wide Web: www.Amednews.com.

Matousek, M. (2007, January and February). We're Wired to Connect. *AARP*, 36–38.

May, R. (1967). The Origins and Significance of the Existential Movement in Psychology. In R. May, E. Angel, and H. Ellenberger (eds.), *Existence: A New Dimension in Psychology*. New York: Simon & Schuster.

McAlister, F. A. (2003). Applying Evidence to Patient Care: from Black and White to Shades of Grey. *Annals of Internal Medicine, 138,* 938–39.

McBeam, E. (1974 [1957]). *The Poisoned Needle*. Mokelumne Hill, CA: Health Research.

McEwen, B., and E. Lasley (2002). *The End of Stress As We Know It*. Washington, DC: Joseph Henry Press.

McKeown, R. E., S. P. Cuffe, and M. Schulz. (2006). U.S. Suicide Rates by Age Group, 1970–2002. *American Journal of Public Health, 96,* 1744–51.

McKinlay, J., and S. McKinlay. (1994). Medical Measures and the Decline of Mortality. In P. Conrad and R. Kern (eds.), *The Sociology of Health & Illness*. Fourth edition. New York: St. Martin's.

McNeill, J. (1932). Medicine for Sin As Prescribed in the Penitentials. *Church History 1,* 14–26.

McNeill, W. (2006). *The Time of Life: Heidegger and Ethos*. Albany, NY: SUNY Press.

McNutt, R. A. (2004). Shared Decision Making. *JAMA, 292,* 2516–18.

Mead, R. (2006, November 13). Proud Flesh, *The New Yorker*, 88–90.

Medical News Today. (2006). Landmark STAR*D Depression Study Offers "Sobering" Third Round Results. Retrieved from the World Wide Web: www.Medicalnewstoday.com/medicalnews.php?newsid=46265.

Menninger, K. (1973). *Whatever Became of Sin?* New York: Hawthorn Press.

Merleau-Ponty, M. (1962). *The Phenomenology of Perception* (C. Smith, trans.). Atlantic Highlands, NJ: Humanities Press.

Metchinkoff, E. (1971 [1939]). *The Founders of Modern Medicine: Pasteur, Koch, Lister*. Freeport, NY: Books for Libraries.

Micale, M. (1993). On the Disappearance of Hysteria: A Study in the Clinical Deconstruction of a Diagnosis. *Isis, 84,* 496–526.

Moalem, S., and J. Prince. (2007). *Survival of the Sickest*. New York: William Morrow.

Moerman, D. (2002). *Meaning, Medicine and the "Placebo Effect."* Cambridge: Cambridge University Press.

Monastersky, R. (2007, December 20). Professors Could Take Performance-Enhancing Drugs for the Mind. *Chronicle of Higher Education*.

Moravec, H. (1988). *Mind Children: The Future of Robot and Human Intelligence*. Cambridge, MA: Harvard University Press.

Morris, D. (1991). *The Culture of Pain*. Berkeley: University of California Press.

———. (2000). *Illness and Culture*. Berkeley: University of California Press.

Moyers, B. (1993). Healing from Within. Part 3 of *Healing and the Mind*. PBS video.

Moynihan, R., I. Heath, and D. Henry. (2002). Selling Sickness: The Pharmaceutical Industry and Disease Mongering. *British Medical Journal, 324,* 886–91.

Narada. (1969 [1889]). Julius Jolly (trans). Delhi, India: Motilal Banarsidas.

Nash, H. (2006). Physical and Health Benefits. Retrieved from the World Wide Web: www.Peteducation.com/article.cfm?cis=o&cat=1491&articleid=638.

Nietzsche, F. (1968 [1954]). On Truth and Lie in the Extra-moral Sense. In W. Kaufmann (ed.), *The Portable Nietzsche.* New York: Viking.

———. (1969). *Towards A Genealogy of Morals* (W. Kaufmann, trans.). New York: Vintage Books.

———. (1974). *The Gay Science* (W. Kaufmann, trans.). New York: Vintage Books.

Nonclercq, M. (1978). Un Chapitre Ignoré de L'Histoire des Sciences: L'ouevre de Béchamp. *Compt. Rend. 103 Cong. Nat. Soc. Savant, 5,* 107–69.

Nores, J. (1999). The Philosophy of Pain. *Journal of Chronic Fatigue Syndrome, 5,* 99–105.

O'Connor, R. (2005). *Undoing Perpetual Stress: The Missing Connection between Depression, Anxiety, and 21st Century Illness.* New York: Berkeley Books.

O'Malley, M. (2005). The Busyness That is Not Business: Nervousness and Character at the Turn of the Last Century. *Social Research, 72,* 371–406.

Ogle, K. (2001, November 6). Sometimes the Doctor is Blind. *New York Times.*

Oransky, I., and S. Savitz. (1998, April 17). Aloof Med Students Lack Empathy for Patients. *USA Today.*

Ornish, D. (1998). *Love & Survival: The Scientific Basis for the Healing Power of Intimacy.* New York: HarperCollins.

Palmer, M. (2006). *Natural Causes: Death, Lies and Politics in America's Vitamin and Herbal Supplement Industry.* New York: Broadway Publishers.

Paumgarten, N. (2007, April 16). There and Back Again. *The New Yorker,* 58–70.

Pearson, R. B. (1942). The Dream and Lie of Louis Pasteur. Retrieved from the World Wide Web: www.whale.to/v/pasteur.

Pennebaker, J. (1997). *Opening Up: The Healing Power of Expressing Emotions.* New York: Guilford Press.

Pert, C. (1999). *The Molecules of Emotion: The Science Behind Mind-Body Medicine.* New York: Scribner's.

Peters, P. (1993). *Warning: Vaccinations Are Dangerous!* LaPorte, CO.: Scriptures for America.

Phillips, K. (1996). *The Broken Mirror.* New York: Oxford University Press.

Plato. (1995) *Phaedrus* (A. Nehamas and P. Woodruff, trans.). Indianapolis: Hackett Publishing Company.

Pogge, R. C. (1963). The Toxic Placebo. *Medical Times, 91,* 778–81.

Popper, K. (1968). *The Logic of Scientific Discovery.* New York: Harper Torchbooks.

Pronger, B. (2002). *Body Fascism: Salvation in the Technology of Physical Fitness.* Toronto, Canada: University of Toronto Press.

Redding, P. (1995). Science, Medicine, and Illness: Rediscovering the Patient as a Person. In P. Komesaroff (ed.), *Troubled Bodies: Critical Perspectives on Postmodernism, Medical Ethics, and the Body.* Durham, NC: Duke University Press.

Reichmanis, M., A. A. Marino, and R. O. Becker. (1979). LaPlace Plane Analysis of Impedance on the H Meridian. *American Journal of Chinese Medicine, 7,* 188–93.

Reynolds, C. F. (2006). Maintenance Treatment of Major Depression in Old Age. *New England Journal of Medicine, 345*, 1130–38.

Richardson, F., B. Fowers, and C. Guignon. (1999). *Re-Envisioning Psychology.* San Francisco: Jossey-Bass.

Rijke, R. P. C. (1985). Cancer and the Development of Will. *Theoretical Medicine, 6*, 133–42.

Ringel, S. P. (2003). Patients Like Linda. *JAMA, 290*, 165–66.

Ritzer, G. (2002). *The McDonaldization of Society.* Thousand Oaks, CA: Sage.

Roach, M. (2003). *Stiff: The Curious Lives of Human Cadavers.* New York: W.W. Norton.

Rosa, H. (2003). Social Acceleration: Ethical and Political Consequences of a Desynchronized High-Speed Society. *Constellations, 10*, 1–33.

Rosenbaum, E. E. (1988). *A Taste of My Own Medicine: When the Doctor is Patient.* New York: Random House.

Rush, A. J., M. H. Trivedi, S. R. Wisniewski, J. W. Stewart, A. A. Nierenberg, M. E. Thase, et al. (2006). Bupropion-SR, Sertraline, or Venlafaxine-XR after Failure of SSRIs for Depression. *New England Journal of Medicine, 354*, 1231–42.

Salon.com. (2000). Germ Theory of Obesity Gains Weight. Retrieved from the World Wide Web: www.archive.salon.com/health/feature/2000/09/19/fat_germ/index.html.

Salyers, A., and D. Whitt. (2005). *Revenge of the Microbes.* Washington, DC: ASM Press.

Sander, A., and V. Colliver. (2004, February 22). Antidepressants Hazardous to Health Care Coverage: Insurance Plans Stymie Individual Policy Holders. *San Francisco Chronicle.*

Sardi, B. (2006, July 26). The Germ Theory of Heart Disease. Retrieved from the World Wide Web: www.Knowledgeofhealth.com.

Sartre, J. (1956). *Being and Nothingness* (H. Barnes, trans.). New York: Washington Square Press.

———. (1989). *No Exit and Three Other Plays* (S. Gilbert, trans.). New York: Vintage International.

Scarry, E. (1985). *The Body in Pain.* New York: Oxford University Press.

Scheler, M. (1958). *The Nature of Sympathy* (Peter Heath, trans.). London: Routledge & Kegan Paul.

Schopenhauer, A. (1965). *On the Basis of Morality* (E. F. J. Payne, trans.). Indianapolis: Library of Liberal Arts.

Schott, R. (1988). *Cognition and Eros.* Boston: Beacon Press.

Sedgwick, P. (1973). Illness, Mental and Otherwise: All Illness Expresses a Social Judgment. *Hastings Center Studies, 1*, 19–40.

Selye, H. (1976). *The Stress of Life.* New York: McGraw-Hill.

Shah, S. (2006). *The Body Hunters.* New York: The New Press.

Shapiro, A. (1960). A Contribution to a History of the Placebo Effect. *Behavioral Science, 5*, 109–35.

Sheehy, G. (2006, June 18). Why Marriage is Good Medicine for Men. *Parade Magazine*, 4–5.

Shlim, D., and N. R. Chokyi. (2006). *Medicine & Compassion*. Boston: Wisdom Pub.

Shorter, E. (1997). *A History of Psychiatry: From the Era of the Asylum to the Age of Prozac*. New York: John Wiley and Sons, Inc.

Showalter, E. (1997). *Hystories*. New York: Columbia University Press.

Sifneos, P. E. (1973). The Prevalence of "Alexithymic" Characteristics in Psychomatic Patients. *Psychotherapy and Psychosomatics, 22*, 255–62.

———. (1996). Alexithemia: Past and Present. *American Journal of Psychiatry, 153*, 137–42.

Silverman, B., and G. Treisman. (2006). Attention-Deficit Disorder at the Crossroads of Cosmetic and Therapeutic Psychiatry. *Johns Hopkins Advanced Studies in Medicine, 6*, 13–15.

Simmel, G. (1977). *The Problems of the Philosophy of History*. (Guy Oakes, trans. and ed.). New York: Free Press.

———. (1997a). On the Psychology of Money. In D. Frisby and M. Featherstone (eds.), *Simmel on Culture*. London: Sage.

———. (1997b). The Metropolis and Mental Life. In D. Frisby and M. Featherstone (eds.), *Simmel on Culture*. London: Sage.

Sinaikin, P. (2006). Bored to Tears? Depression and Heidegger's Concept of Profound Boredom. Unpublished manuscript.

Skinner, B. F. (1971). *Beyond Freedom and Dignity*. New York: Alfred Knopf.

Sloan, R. P., E. Baglella, and T. Powell. (1999). Religion, Spirituality, and Medicine. *The Lancet, 353*, 664–67.

Smith, J. (1999). *Where the Roots Reach for Water: A Personal and Natural History of Melancholia*. New York: North Point Press.

Smith, T. (2005). Why Isn't the Germ Theory a "Religion"? Retrieved from the World Wide Web: www.pandas thumb.org/archives/2005/07/why_isn't_ge_1.html.

Smith, T. W., and N. B. Anderson. (1986). Models of Personality and Disease: An Interactional Approach to Type A Behavior and Cardiovascular Risk. *Journal of Personality and Social Psychology, 50*, 1166–73.

Sones, B., and R. Sones. (2006, February 15–25). Strange but True. *This Week*.

Sontag, Susan. (1978). *Illness As Metaphor*. New York: Farrar, Straus, and Giroux.

Spacks, Patricia. (1995). *Boredom: The Literary History of a State of Mind*. Chicago: University of Chicago Press.

Specter, M. (2004, February 2). Miracle in a Bottle. *The New Yorker*, 64–75.

———. (2007, March 12). The Denialists. *The New Yorker*, 32–38.

Spiegel, A. (2005, January 3). The Dictionary of Disorder. *The New Yorker*, 56–63.

Spiegel, D., J. R. Bloom, H. C. Kraemer, and E. Gottheil. (1989, October 14). Effect of Psychosocial Treatment on Survival of Patients with Metastatic Breast Cancer. *The Lancet, 2 (8668)*, 888–91.

Spiegel, D., and M. Cordova. (2001). Supportive-Expressive Group Therapy and Life Extension of Breast Cancer Patients. *Advances in Mind-Body Medicine, 17*, 38–41.

Sprenger, J., and H. Krämer. (1970 [1486]). *Malleus Malificorum (Hammer of Witches)* (M. Sumers, trans.). New York: Benjamin Blom.

Starr, P. (1982). *The Social Transformation of American Medicine.* New York: Basic Books.

Stein, E. (1964). *On the Problem of Empathy* (W. Stein, trans.). The Hague: Martinus Nijhoff.

Stein, M. (2007). *The Lonely Patient: How We Experience Illness.* New York: HarperCollins.

Sudnow, D. (1967). *Passing On.* Englewood Cliffs, NJ: Prentice-Hall.

Svenaeus, F. (2000). *The Hermeneutics of Medicine and the Phenomenology of Health.* Boston: Kluwer Academic Pub.

Szasz, T. (1965). *Psychiatric Justice.* New York: Macmillan.

———. (1970). *The Manufacture of Madness.* New York: Dell Publishing.

———. (1971). The Sane Slave: An Historical Note on the Use of Medical Diagnosis as Justificatory Rhetoric. *American Journal of Psychiatry, 25*, 228–39.

———. (1974). *The Myth of Mental Illness.* New York: Harper & Row.

———. (1975). *Ceremonial Chemistry: The Ritual Persecution of Drugs, Addicts, and Pushers.* New York: Anchor-Doubleday.

Taylor, G. J. (1984). Alexithymia: Concept, Measurement and Implications for Treatment. *American Journal of Psychiatry, 141*, 725–32.

———. (1991). The Alexithymia Construct: A Potential Paradigm for Psychosomatic Medicine. *Psychosomatics, 32*, 153–64.

Tempkin, O. (1977). *The Double Face of Janus.* Baltimore: Johns Hopkins University Press.

Thomas, W. I. (1969). *On Social Organization and Social Personality.* Chicago: University of Chicago Press.

Tolstoy, L. (1960). *The Death of Ivan Ilych and Other Short Stories.* New York: The New American Library.

Tönnies, F. (1957). *Community and Society* (C. Loomis, trans.). Lansing: Michigan State University Press.

Toombs, S. K. (1992). *The Meaning of Illness: A Phenomenological Account of the Different Perspectives of Physician and Patient.* Boston: Kluwer Academic Pub.

Trivedi, M., M. Fava, S. R. Wisniewski, M. E. Thas, F. Quitkin, et al. (2006). Medication Augmentation after the Failure of SSRIs for Depression. *New England Journal of Medicine, 354*, 1243–51.

Ullman, D. (1995). A Homeopathic Perspective on AIDS. Retrieved from the World Wide Web: www.homeopathic.com/articles/using_h/aids.php.

Ulmer, D. K., and L. Schwartzburd. (1996). Treatment of Time Pathologies. In *Heart and Mind: The Practice of Cardiac Psychology.* Washington, DC: American Psychological Association.

Verrengia, J. B. (2005, March 20). Modern Home Life Is Always in Motion. *Idaho State Journal*.

Waitzkin, H. (1994). A Marxian Interpretation of the Growth and Development of Coronary Care Technology. In P. Conrad and R. Kern (eds.), *The Sociology of Health & Illness: Critical Perspectives*. Fourth edition. New York: St. Martin's Press.

Weber, M. (1946). Politics as a Vocation. In H. Gerth and C. W. Mills (eds.), *From Max Weber*. New York: Oxford University Press.

———. (1958). *The Protestant Ethic and the Spirit of Capitalism* (T. Parsons, trans.). New York: Charles Scribner's Sons.

Weeks, J. (1991). Sexual Identification is A Strange Thing. In *Against Nature: Essays on History, Sexuality and Identity*. London: Oram Press.

Wendell, S. (1996). *The Rejected Body: Feminist Philosophical Reflection on Disability*. New York: Routledge.

Whorf, B. (1956). *Language, Thought, and Reality*. Cambridge, MA: Massachusetts Institute of Technology.

Williams, M., J. Teasdale, Z. Segal, and J. Kabat-Zinn. (2007). *The Mindful Way through Depression: Freeing Yourself from Chronic Unhappiness*. New York and London: The Guilford Press.

Willing, R. (1999, April 26). Study: Worshippers Live Longer Than Those Who Skip Services. *USA Today*.

Wilson, R. (1968). *Feminine Forever*. N.p.: M. Evans and Co., Inc.

Wolbring, G. (2006). The Enhancement Debate: or Able-ism Leads to Transhumanism. Unpublished address given to the James Martin Institute for Science and Civilisation. Said Business School, University of Oxford, England.

Wolf, S., and H. Wolff. (1947). *Human Gastric Function*. New York: Oxford University Press.

Woods, D. R., and T. Cagney. (1993). Clinician Update: The Nuts and Bolts of Managing Managed Care. *Behavioral Healthcare Tomorrow, 2*, 38–39.

Xenophilia. (2003). The Rife Microscope Story. Retrieved from the World Wide Web: www.xenophilia.com/zb/zb0012.

Yalom, I. (1980). *Existential Psychotherapy*. New York: HarperCollins.

Young, I. M. (1990). *Throwing Like a Girl and Other Essays in Feminist Philosophy and Social Theory*. Bloomington: Indiana University Press.

———. (2005). *On Female Body Experience*. New York: Oxford University Press.

Zaner, R. (1981). *The Context of Self*. Athens, OH: Ohio University Press.

———. (1984). The Phenomenon of Medicine: Of Hoaxes and Humor. In D. H. Brock and A. Harvard (eds.), *The Culture of Biomedicine*. London: Associated University Presses.

———. (2004). *Conversations on the Edge: Narratives of Ethics and Illness*. Washington, DC: Georgetown University Press.

Zborowski, M. (1969). *People in Pain*. San Francisco: Jossey-Bass.

Zerubavel, E. (2006). *Elephant in the Room*. New York: Oxford University Press.

Index

MAY - - 2012